HANS POPPER
A Tribute

HANS POPPER

A Tribute

Editors

Paul D. Berk, M.D.
Division of Liver Diseases
The Mount Sinai School of Medicine
New York, New York

Fenton Schaffner, M.D.
Division of Liver Diseases
The Mount Sinai School of Medicine
New York, New York

Rudi Schmid, M.D.
Department of Medicine
University of California
San Francisco, California

RAVEN PRESS ⬥ NEW YORK

Raven Press, Ltd., 1185 Avenue of the Americas, New York, New York 10036

Made in the United States of America

Library of Congress Cataloging-in-Publication Data

Hans Popper : a tribute / editors, Paul D. Berk, Fenton Schaffner,
   Rudi Schmid.
         p.   cm.
   Includes bibliographical references and index.
   ISBN 0-88167-833-3
   1. Liver—Diseases. 2. Popper, Hans, 1903– . I. Berk, Paul D.
II. Schaffner. Fenton, 1920– . III. Schmid, Rudi, 1922– .
   [DNLM: 1. Popper, Hans, 1903– . 2. Gastroenterology—biography.
3. Liver Diseases—essays. WI 700 H249]
RC845.H37 1991
616.3′62—dc20
DNLM/DLC
for Library of Congress   91-27884
                                                    CIP

9 8 7 6 5 4 3 2 1

Contents

Contributors

George Acs
Department of Biochemistry, The Mount Sinai School of Medicine, Box 1020, 1 Gustave L. Levy Place, New York, New York 10029

Irwin M. Arias
Department of Physiology, Tufts University School of Medicine, 136 Harrison Avenue, Boston, Massachusetts 02111

Paul D. Berk
Division of Liver Diseases, The Mount Sinai School of Medicine, Box 1039, 1 Gustave L. Levy Place, New York, New York 10029

Leonardo Bianchi
Institut für Pathologie der Universität Basel, Schönbeinstrasse 40, CH-4003 Basel/Schweiz, Switzerland

Baruch S. Blumberg
Fox Chase Cancer Center, 7701 Burholme Avenue, Philadelphia, Pennsylvania 19111

James L. Boyer
Liver Study Unit, Department of Internal Medicine, Yale University, 333 Cedar Street, New Haven, Connecticut 06510

Nijole Brazenas
Department of Pathology, St. Joseph Medical Center, 127 South Broadway, Yonkers, New York 10701

Thomas C. Chalmers
Technology Assessment Group, Harvard School of Public Health, Room L-7A, 677 Huntington Avenue, Boston, Massachusetts 02115

Whan Kook Chung
Catholic University Medical College, Catholic Medical Center, 62, Youido-Dong, Youngdeungpo-Gu, Seoul, Korea

Harold O. Conn
Department of Internal Medicine, Liver Disease Unit (111E), Yale University, Veterans Administration Medical Center, West Spring Street, New Haven, Connecticut 06516

W. Graham E. Cooksley
Clinical Research Centre, Royal Brisbane Hospital Foundation, The Bancroft Centre, 300 Herston Road, Brisbane, Q.4029, P.O. Royal Brisbane Hospital, Brisbane, Australia 4029

Helmut Denk
Pathologisches Institut der Universität Graz, Auenbrugger Platz 25, A-8036 Graz, Austria

V. J. Desmet
Universitair Ziekenhuisen Leuven, Sint Rafael, Patholog. Ontleedkunde B, Minderbroedersstraat 12, B-3000 Leuven, Belgium

Herbert Falk
Falk Foundation, Leinenweberstrasse 5, D-7800 Freiburg im Breisgau, Germany

Stephen A. Geller
Cedars-Sinai Medical Center, 8700 Beverly Boulevard, Los Angeles, California 90048-1869

Michael A. Gerber
Department of Pathology, Tulane University Medical Center, 1430 Tulane Avenue, New Orleans, Louisiana 70112

John L. Gerin
Division of Molecular Virology and Immunology, Georgetown University, 5640 Fishers Lane, Rockville, Maryland 20852

Wolfgang Gerok
Medizinische Klinik der Universität Freiburg, Hugstetter Strasse 55, D-7800 Freiburg im Breisgau, Germany

Helmut Greim
GSF-Forschungszentrum für Umwelt und Gesundheit, Institut für Toxikologie, Ingolstädter Landstrasse 1, D-8042 Neuherberg, Germany

Pauline Hall
Department of Histopathology, Flinders Medical Centre, Bedford Park 5042, South Australia

June W. Halliday
Queensland Institute of Medical Research (Liver Program), The Bancroft Centre, 300 Herston Road, Brisbane, Q.4029, P.O. Royal Brisbane Hospital, Brisbane, Australia 4029

Kamal G. Ishak
Department of Hepatic Pathology, Armed Forces Institute of Pathology, Washington, DC 20306

Sarah C. Kalser
National Institute of Diabetes and Digestive and Kidney Diseases (NIDDK), Westwood Building, Room 3A17, 5333 Westbard Avenue, Bethesda, Maryland 20892

Donald King
University of Chicago, 5841 South Maryland Avenue, Chicago, Illinois 62637

Sherman Kupfer
Department of Medicine, The Mount Sinai School of Medicine, Box 1027, 1 Gustave L. Levy Place, New York, New York 10029

Karoly Lapis
I. Institute of Pathology and Experimental Cancer Research, Semmelweis Medical University, 1085 Budapest VIII, Ulloi ut 26, Hungary

Carroll M. Leevy
Department of Medicine, University of Medicine and Dentistry of New Jersey, University Heights, 185 South Orange Avenue, Newark, New Jersey 07103-2714

Jay H. Lefkowitch
Department of Pathology, College of Physicians and Surgeons of Columbia University, 630 West 168th Street, New York, New York 10032

Charles S. Lieber
Alcohol Research and Treatment Center, Liver Disease and Nutrition Section, Bronx Veterans Administration Medical Center, 130 West Kingsbridge Road, Bronx, New York 10468

Ian R. Mackay
Centre for Molecular Biology and Medicine, Monash University, Clayton, Victoria 3168, Australia

M.P. MacSween
Department of Pathology, University of Glasgow, Western Infirmary, Glasgow G11 6NT, United Kingdom

R.N.M. MacSween
Department of Pathology, University of Glasgow, Western Infirmary, Glasgow G11 6NT, United Kingdom

Reba Kasten Nosoff
Sloane Hospital for Women, Columbia-Presbyterian Medical Center, New York, New York 10032-3784

Kunio Okuda
First Department of Internal Medicine, Chiba University School of Medicine, 1-8-1, Inohana, Chiba City 280, Japan

Fiorenzo Paronetto
Department of Pathology, Bronx Veterans Administration Medical Center, 130 West Kingsbridge Road, Bronx, New York 10468

Victor Perez
Facultad de Medicina, Universidad de Buenos Aires and Division de Gastroenterologia, Hospital Escuela Jose de San Martin, M.T. de Alvear 2346, 1122 Buenos Aires, Argentina

Lawrie W. Powell
Queensland Institute of Medical Research (Liver Program), The Bancroft Centre, 300 Herston Road, Brisbane, Q.4029, P.O. Royal Brisbane Hospital, Brisbane, Australia 4029

Robert H. Purcell
Hepatitis Viruses Section, National Institutes of Health, Building 7, Room 202, 9000 Rockville Pike, Bethesda, Maryland 20892

Marcus A. Rothschild
Nuclear Medicine Service/115, Veterans Administration Medical Center, First Avenue at East 24th Street, New York, New York 10010

William Rutter
Hormone Research Institute, University of California at San Francisco, 1098 HSW, San Francisco, California 94143-0534

Fenton Schaffner
Division of Liver Diseases, The Mount Sinai School of Medicine, Box 1101, 1 Gustave L. Levy Place, New York, New York 10029

Peter J. Scheuer
Royal Free Hospital School of Medicine, University of London, Pond Street, London NW3 2QG, United Kingdom

Steven Schenker
Division of Gastroenterology, University of Texas Health Sciences Center, 7703 Floyd Curl Drive, San Antonio, Texas 78284

Rudi Schmid
Department of Medicine, University of California, 1120 HSW, GI Unit, San Francisco, California 94143

Thomas E. Starzl
Department of Surgery, University of Pittsburgh School of Medicine, 3601 Fifth Avenue, Pittsburgh, Pennsylvania 15213

Frederick Steigmann
1205 West Kirby Avenue, Champaign, Illinois 61821

Heribert Thaler
Sebastianplatz 7/5, A-1030 Wien, Austria

Swan N. Thung
The Lillian and Henry M. Stratton-Hans Popper Department of Pathology, The Mount Sinai School of Medicine, 1 Gustave L. Levy Place, New York, New York 10029

Hyman J. Zimmerman
Armed Forces Institute of Pathology, Center for Special Studies in Hepatotoxicity, Washington, DC 20306-6000

INTRODUCTION

Paul D. Berk, New York

Hans Popper, father of the modern discipline of hepatology, founder of the American Association for the Study of Liver Diseases (AASLD) and the International Association for the Study of the Liver (IASL), moving force behind the creation of The Mount Sinai School of Medicine, role model for three generations of clinical scientists, and my mentor and friend, died in New York of pancreatic carcinoma on May 6, 1988, just 6 months short of his 85th birthday. In the year that followed his passing, his remarkable life and innumerable contributions to science and medicine were recalled in editorials in many prominent journals and in a special issue of *Seminars in Liver Disease*. He was also memorialized during a day-long symposium at The Mount Sinai School of Medicine, to which he had devoted much of his energy over the last 21 years of his life. At this symposium, distinguished scientists from around the world described the current state of the art in their respective disciplines and predicted directions of future progress in areas central to the scientific basis of hepatology. It was a day Hans would have thoroughly enjoyed, not the least because every speaker was able to point out some new way in which Hans' own insights had altered the direction of research and progress in his field. Both the symposium at Mount Sinai and the memorial issue of *Seminars in Liver Disease* focused on basic science, often in its most fundamental aspects. In this regard, they reflected the in-

This remembrance of Hans is expanded from one which appeared as a Foreword in the November 1988 issue of *Seminars in Liver Disease*. It is printed here with the kind permission of Thieme Medical Publishers, Inc.

1

creasingly basic evolution of Hans' own interests and his abiding conviction that the future of clinical progress lay in the basic science laboratory.

The essential features of Hans' curriculum vitae are well known. He was born in Vienna in 1903, the only son of Emma Gruenbaum and Dr. Karl Popper, a distinguished Viennese physician. Hans began his medical studies at the University of Vienna at the age of 19, training in chemistry and conducting his initial research in the new but blossoming field of biochemistry. Among his early accomplishments was the development of the creatinine clearance as a quantitative test of renal function.

In 1938, warned of his imminent arrest by the Nazis, he fled his native Austria and settled in Chicago, where he was the recipient of a research fellowship at Cook County Hospital. Within a few short years, he assembled there a distinguished hepatic research group and was the principal force behind the creation of the renowned Hektoen Institute for Medical Research. He eventually became the director of pathology at Cook County, where, with his younger associate, Dr. Fenton Schaffner, he wrote the first modern textbook in the English language on the pathology of the liver. His Chicago days also saw the founding of AASLD, which grew out of meetings initially held at the Hektoen Institute, and of IASL.

In 1957, Hans was enticed from Chicago to the post of pathologist-in-chief at The Mount Sinai Hospital in New York. He was among the first to perceive that, in the biomedical environment of the time, Mount Sinai would need a medical school if its 125-year tradition of clinical and intellectual excellence was to continue to thrive. Persuasive as always, he brought the board of trustees around to his point of view; the Mount Sinai School of Medicine was formally established in 1963. Hans was its first dean for academic affairs. He was also the first chairman of its Department of Pathology and the first Irene Heinz Given and John LaPorte Given Professor of Pathology. Since 1985, as the result of the generosity of Hans' late friend, the prominent medical publisher Henry M. Stratton, the department has been designated the Lillian and Henry Stratton-Hans Popper Department of Pathology. Hans served in 1972–1973 in the joint posts of dean of the Mount Sinai School of Medicine and president of the Mount Sinai Medical Center. He retired from formal administrative obligations in 1973, but, as a Gustave L. Levy Distinguished Service Professor, remained an active member of the faculty until his death.

The emphasis here should certainly be on the word "active." Hans worked a 7-day week well into his ninth decade; until just weeks before his death, his work day ended long after mere mortals had gone home and supped. His incredible ability to see associations between studies in seemingly disparate fields and to make connections that had eluded others were the result, certainly, of his genius but also of his incredible capacity and enthusiasm for hard work. To the very end, no newly received journal reached the shelves of the library at Mount Sinai without an overnight stay in Hans' office, where it was perused, digested, and anything of interest integrated into his already vast store of knowledge. He never went to sleep at night, he once told me, without asking himself two questions: "What did I learn today? What gave me joy today?" Unique among men, he had a positive answer for both questions every day of his life.

Hans' research encompassed virtually every area of hepatology. He was especially proud of his ability to understand processes at the molecular level based on observations with the light microscope and hematoxylin-and-eosin-stained tissue sections. His insights over his last decade into the pathobiology of viral hepatitis were truly remarkable. At the time of his death, he was working on a unified hypothesis concerning the molecular basis for hepatocellular carcinogenesis that accounted for differences between chemically induced and virally induced hepatic neoplasms.

I first met Hans in the fall of 1961. The Mount Sinai School of Medicine had not yet come into being, and as professor of pathology at Columbia's College of Physicians and Surgeons, where I was a second-year student, he gave an extraordinary series of lectures on the pathology of the liver. Their brilliance was only slightly obscured by his accent, which was somewhat thicker then than later in his life. With the impertinence of which only second-year medical students are capable, he was petitioned to give his lectures in German, on the hypothesis that then at least the handful of German speakers in the class would fully understand him and could prepare a set of lecture notes for the others. As unelected class fool, I was somehow designated to present him with the proposition. He listened patiently and politely, then lapsed into thought for several minutes, all the while, so it seemed to me, staring intently at my name tag while I profoundly prayed for some form of divine intervention that would allow me to vanish in a puff of smoke. At last he spoke. "You know," he said, "I am an educator as well as physician. It is well known that American medical students are woefully deficient in their command of their native language. As an educator, it would be wrong to pander to this deficiency. For the sake of your own education, I will continue to lecture in English." It was more than a decade before Hans and I were again alone together in a room. I was by then chief of the Section on Diseases of the Liver at the National Institutes of Health (NIH) in Bethesda; he, having recently arrived as a Fogarty Scholar in Residence, had been guest speaker at our weekly noon conference. I had found his talk stimulating and provocative and, as was the custom at those conferences, I and others had interrupted him frequently with questions. Then, with the meeting over and the rest of the audience having left, he approached me in the rear of the room. A smile of recognition appeared surprisingly on his face, and he extended his hand in greeting. "It's good to see you again," he said. "And I'm glad your English has finally improved." His incredible memory, his sense of humor, and his extraordinary interest in young people were never more evident nor more appreciated.

The Washington/Bethesda metropolitan area to which Hans came for his Fogarty years already constituted a unique hepatologic community. Physicians and scientists with an interest in the liver from all of the area's many scientific and academic institutions—including NIH, Georgetown and George Washington Universities, the Armed Forces Institute of Pathology (AFIP), the Washington Veterans Administration Medical Center, Walter Reed Army Medical Center, and the National Naval Medical Center—worked together as a harmonious and cooperative intellectual community, with a lack of interinstitutional rivalry such as I have never seen in any other city before or since. In addition to innumerable collaborations on specific research projects and clinical trials, the intellectual life of this unique community of scholars was stimulated by two important activities: the bi-weekly Washington Inter-Institutional Journal Club and a weekly liver biopsy conference held at the AFIP.

The Journal Club had been founded some years earlier by Hy Zimmerman and Tom Chalmers, and its evening meetings initially alternated between their respective homes. Everyone, from junior fellow to department chairman, was welcome, the only proviso being that there were no spectators. If you wanted to come, you had to participate by reporting regularly on articles of interest that had appeared in a group of journals assigned to you. Frankie Chalmers and Kitty Zimmerman were exceptionally gracious hostesses, and the camaraderie and scientific exchange in those early days were accompanied by an impressive array of home-baked cookies, chocolate brownies, and other goodies. Even the family dogs participated: one of the Chalmers' beautiful red Irish setters, ordinarily as frisky as a puppy, would sit quietly at my feet in front of the fire and take in the discussions. Shortly before Hans' arrival as a Fogarty Scholar, the growing membership of the Journal Club forced a change of venue to a conference room at NIH. Although the ambience there was less cozy, the intellectual atmosphere remained as charged and stimulating as ever.

The second key activity was the weekly liver biopsy conference at AFIP, presided over by Kamal Ishak, with Hy Zimmerman as senior clinician. Lionel Rabin from AFIP, Leonard Seeff from the VA Hospital, Leonard Goldstein, then at Fort Belvoir, and Tony Jones and I from NIH were among the hard core regulars who, along with a changing cadre of fellows and any invited visitors, gathered around the multi-headed teaching microscopes to review the slides of fascinating cases submitted to AFIP from all over the world for Kamal's review. All cases were initially examined as unknowns; after making a histologic interpretation, Dr. Zimmerman would also attempt to predict the clinical history before Drs. Ishak or Rabin filled us in on the available clinical data. As with the Journal Club, the liver biopsy conference was stimulating and enjoyable and had become a well-established Washington tradition.

It was to this organized and smoothly functioning community that Hans Popper moved in 1974. His impending arrival was, in fact, the cause for mixed emotions. We all knew of Hans Popper. Who didn't? But while a number of us even knew him personally, none of us felt we knew him well. Tom Chalmers, who knew him best, had just moved to Mount Sinai as president and dean, replacing Hans in these posts. This move, engineered by Popper, was precisely what freed him of his administrative responsibilities in New York, so that he could come to the Fogarty Center in Washington. None of us doubted Hans' brilliance or that we all had much to learn from him. There was concern, though, about how this man, who loomed larger than life over every meeting he attended and seemed to dominate our entire discipline, would interact with us and impact on our cozy and established institutions and traditions.

We need not have worried. Within the restricted world of Washington hepatology, Hans moved as if on tip-toes, initially watching, listening, and taking it all in. As he got to know the local players, with many of whom he and Lina initiated or strengthened exceptionally cordial friendships, he began to contribute as well, but always in a manner that displayed extraordinary sensitivity to the feelings of the "locals." He displayed a unique gift for enlivening a discussion, solving a problem, unraveling a mystery, or stimulating an ongoing investigation without in any way dominating or overriding his colleagues. Whatever apprehensions we may have had gave way to a sense of great good fortune on our part to have had this remarkable visitor with us.

Watching Hans in action in virtually any sphere was truly an education. To me, perhaps the most striking recollections are of the AFIP conferences and of the different styles with which Hans and Kamal Ishak approached the interpretation of a complex unknown specimen. Kamal worked logically, methodically, systematically. He would first describe the abnormal histopathologic features he saw, formulate a differential diagnosis, and then, entity by entity, consider all of the possibilities before arriving at a final conclusion. When he finally arrived at a diagnosis, it was by means of a set of explicit thought processes that had been laid out for all to follow. Given the same slide to read again at a later time, his analysis was virtually 100% reproducible. He was almost never wrong. By contrast, Hans would look at a slide quickly and, after what seemed like a nanosecond, or at most a millisecond, arrive at a diagnosis. His conclusions were also virtually almost always right; in fact, he and Kamal rarely disagreed. But in contrast to Ishak, who clearly arrived at his conclusions by a reproducible, logical approach, Hans seemed to work by a unique mechanism that may either have been an exceptional intuition or an equally unique process of pattern recognition based on his long and vast experience. Although his accuracy was astonishing, he sometimes could not explain precisely how he had arrived at a particular conclusion.

Hans' productivity was truly amazing. He was the author of almost 800 articles and author or editor of 28 books. The subset of these publications that appeared after his retirement from his administrative posts at age 70 exceeded by far the output of most lifetimes. Of his numerous achievements, he was proudest of his role in founding The Mount Sinai School of Medicine and of his establishment of two endowed chairs there, and of the success of his many trainees, who are the chairmen of numerous Departments of Pathology around the world and who hold two of the three endowed chairs of pathology in his native Austria. Hans was a member of four major academies, including the National Academy of Sciences of the United States of America and the American Academy of Arts and Sciences, as well as the recipient of 14 honorary doctorates, including one awarded by the University of Vienna at the celebration of the 600th anniversary of its founding. He was also honored by the creation of the International Hans Popper Award, as well as the Hans Popper Förderpreis for the best work on liver disease by a young scientist published in the German language, both granted every 3 years by the Falk Foundation on the occasion of Basel Liver Week; and of the Hans Popper Liver Scholar Endowment Fund, through which the American Liver Foundation supports promising young investigators in the field of hepatic pathobiology and disease. Hans is survived by two sons: Frank, Chairman of the Department of Urban Studies at Rutgers University, and Charles, a child psychiatrist and psychopharmacologist at Harvard. He is also survived by his wife, Lina, to whose patience, wisdom, and support he repeatedly credited his success. His life enriched all who knew him.

1

George Acs, New York

I knew Hans Popper for only a decade, but my respect for him was as deep as if we had known each other for a lifetime. When we met, we immediately re-established the Austria-Hungary monarchy within Mount Sinai with the traditional leadership and supremacy of Austria. The basis of our relationship was that I was a molecular biologist who had started to work with hepatitis B, and, for Hans, the liver was not the most important thing, it was the only thing (paraphrased). To use his own words: "The progress in cellular and molecular biology and the new wonder world of techniques may help us reach the ultimate goal of hepatology—a rational therapy for the basic phenomena and, with it, of the common liver diseases."

Hans Popper was born in an era characterized, with slight exaggeration, by a French comedy in the following way: "Today we shall bleed all those on the left side of the ward and give a purgative to all those on the right side."

Dr. Popper deserves the lion's share of credit for the level of sophistication the field of hepatology has achieved. He was a highly successful scientist who did not desert the laboratory bench. He would sacrifice anything but his beloved microscope, which was not only a physical but also a spiritual extension of his eyes and brain. His life and work, which were inseparable, were testimony to Pasteur's words: "In the field of observation, chance favors the mind that is prepared." Dr. Popper realized that the world of science offered life's greatest opportunities to serve humanity and, at the same time, some of its greatest compensations. The pursuit of science gives happiness; I suspect that only a few scientists enjoyed their work as much as Dr. Popper.

Many scientific papers seem very important when they appear, but as the field develops, it is apparent that they are less significant than was first thought. As time goes on, truly significant contributions become lasting landmarks. Many of Dr. Popper's papers and contributions are an example. Personally, I can only repeat:

> It was a great privilege to sit in his office—the walls covered with honorary degrees—watching him pace back and forth with olympic speed thinking aloud. When a new idea occurred to him, it was always accompanied by a big grin, a twinkle in his eye, and great satisfaction radiated from his face. . . . In remembering Dr. Hans Popper, one has to mention his wife, Lina, an exceptional woman who stood beside him for a lifetime. She encouraged him, served as an intellectual stimulus and, with charm and grace, protected him from enemies, friends and himself.

It is unfair that he cannot see and contribute to further developments. I am one of the many fortunate people who received inspiration and guidance from him. I am convinced that future generations of hepatologists will receive similar benefits when they read his papers.

2

Irwin M. Arias, Boston

Hans and I shared the editorship of two books and one journal (*Hepatology*) but never published a scientific paper together. Nevertheless, he influenced my professional and personal career in important and innumerable ways. He was my scientific sounding board, "best friend, severest critic," and wise counselor.

We first met during the early days of bilirubin glucuronide research, circa 1955. I was an instructor at the Albert Einstein College of Medicine and had just presented a paper at the Young Turks' meeting in Atlantic City regarding the mechanism of bilirubin glucuronide formation *in vitro*. Two days later, I received a friendly letter of congratulations that included reprints of Hans' early work on glucuronides and a generous invitation to visit his laboratory. I called, arranged an appointment, and spent 2 marvelous hours talking about many aspects of hepatic science, particularly his perception of the increasing need for "modern" biochemical studies in hepatology. From that day, we shared uninhibited and wide-ranging discussions of science, politics, literature, and family. Hans was already a global leader in hepatology at that time. His impact on a young academic physician was enormous and sustained.

To me, Hans' most amazing characteristic was his insatiable desire to learn more about everything, particularly as it might relate to the liver. The older he became, the stronger seemed the urge. Most men and women over the age of 35 spend considerable energy defending their earlier scientific accomplishments. Although Hans relished reference to his early works in chemistry and pathology, he was never defensive. His boundless energy drove him to learn the latest about biochemistry, immunology, cell biology, and molecular biology as each discipline grew from the 1950s to the present. He did not consider himself a basic scientist but stressed the necessity of sustained study to link basic science and human disease, particularly of the liver.

He was very pleased when his three co-editors (Dave Schachter, Dave Shafritz, and myself) of the first edition of *The Liver: Biology and Pathobiology* conspired to dedicate the book to him as follows: "His intellect has inspired and stimulated at least three generations of hepatologists. His broad range of interest and sustained desire to bridge the gap between advances in basic biology and liver structure, function and disease exemplify the purpose of this book."

Through the 1960s, we regularly discussed biochemical work that my colleagues and I were engaged in relating to membrane composition and protein turnover. Hans was, once again, ahead of the times and suggested that membranes must contain molecules that recognize hormones and other signals. He wondered if such molecules had more rapid turnover than did other membrane components. One discussion concerned why bilirubin, bile acids, and other organic compounds selectively enter the liver cell but do not appear to compete with one another. Hans' view was that the plasma membrane must have different special molecules (now called receptors) for each class of substance. Our experiments, which led to the identification of Y and Z as two intracellular organic anion binding proteins, partially resulted from these conversations. He argued persuasively that neither of these proteins could serve as a true "receptor" because they were soluble. Subsequent recognition of soluble hormone receptors that target ligands to the nucleus prompted another conversation in which membrane specificity was downplayed and cytosolic receptors were, as he would frequently say, "the key." Of course, he wasn't always right, but his ideas were novel, ahead of their time, and based on a wealth of information from many disciplines.

Our best discussions concerned the view that intrahepatic cholestasis probably results from hepatocellular abnormalities rather than extracellular obstruction. As evidence in support of the former accumulated, Hans changed his views but consistently asked: "If the defect is hepatocellular, why is the canaliculus dilated in intrahepatic cholestasis?" We still don't know. He was thrilled with Keppler's observation that edema-producing leukotrienes are excreted in the bile. At last, a plausible explanation for canalicular obstruction secondary to a hepatocellular defect was available. I suspect that when we finally unravel the mysteries of vasoactive compounds excreted in bile and associate them with cholestasis, Hans would have said, "Good work . . . but remember that the H-and-E stained sections also suggested an obstructive element."

During most of the 1970s and 1980s, Hans regularly visited the Liver

Research Center at Albert Einstein, where he participated in seminars and exposed us to his amazing Sherlock Holmesian skill of analyzing a case from an H-and-E slide sans history. The few mistakes in diagnosis were as informative as the large number of correct diagnoses. I remember an aspiration liver biopsy from a young woman. The pathology was multiple granulomas. Our experienced pathologists spent about 2 weeks doing special stains trying to exclude sarcoidosis. Hans looked at the projected slide. He quickly said, "This isn't tuberculosis or sarcoid. I haven't seen anything like it." He described his reasons in detail. The diagnosis was leprosy of the liver. Later that year, I visited another institution where Hans had been 2 weeks previously. My colleagues were still amazed at his brilliant diagnosis and discussion of another case of hepatic granuloma in a young woman! The diagnosis was also leprosy! He rarely, if ever, forgot a case. In pathology, as in other areas of science, he built on knowledge and experience. He was a marvelous architect of ideas.

Hans presided over the birth of *Hepatology*. He contributed substantially by helping me to organize the new journal, attract good manuscripts, recruit outstanding basic scientists, and convince skeptics who had doubts about the journal's longevity. As *Hepatology* grew, he and I engaged in a friendly competition to attract outstanding basic scientists who were not hepatologists but whose work should be of interest to the readers. This activity prompted more phone calls, meetings, and evening discussions in the celebrated "liver temple," which was his office at The Mount Sinai Hospital. As with discovery in science or other exciting developments, *Hepatology*'s success gave him great pleasure. He continuously offered suggestions, criticisms, and support, particularly when they were most needed.

In 1984, I was offered an unusual position at Tufts University School of Medicine, as chairman of the Department of Physiology, which could be developed into a major pathophysiology center. The prospect of leaving my academic home at Albert Einstein, where I had been for almost 30 years and had participated in the development of the Liver Research Center, made me anxious. Hans sensed this conflict and other problems of which he was aware. He called and we talked for hours . . . on the phone and in his office. He explored all of my concerns and some of his. He told me personal things that were of help. In the end, when I decided to take on the new challenge, he congratulated me and, to the year of his death, sustained close contact and interest in our educational experiment. Hans met our graduate students and postdoctoral fellows every year. His visit was a highlight of our course in pathophysiology for graduate students. Several students communicated with him for further information, and he provided great support for our program to create basic scientists who are knowledgeable about human diseases.

In 1985, I was a Fogarty Scholar at NIH as Hans had been several years previously. During my tenure at NIH, Hans and I shared many evenings and flights to and from Boston. We exchanged copies of interesting manuscripts from nonhepatologic sources. It was then that I learned how he managed to keep ahead of everyone in knowledge of advances in basic science! Every major journal arriving at the Mount Sinai library came to him for 24 hours, which was sufficient time for him to read, copy, and learn before returning the journal to the library. It still amazes me that he could read so much, be critical and constructive, and remember details, even in fields in which he lacked formal training.

One day we discussed a seminar I had just heard by Mark Willingham of NCI on multidrug resistance, in particular, mdr genes and their 170 Kd protein product. While a Fogarty Fellow at NIH, I obtained human liver, and we observed that Gpl70 is a normal substituent of the bile canaliculus, proximal tubular brush border, and secretory surfaces of other cells. What was this membrane protein, which we later showed is an ATP-requiring transporter, doing in the secretory domains of the plasma membrane of these polarized cells? Two hypotheses seemed possible: (1) Gpl70 has a natural substrate and is merely co-opted by many anti-cancer drugs and other compounds that can be transported by this system. (2) Gpl70 is part of the general detoxification system. Like the p450, GSH transferase, and glucuronyl transferases families of detoxification enzymes, Gpl70 has low affinity but great capacity for ligands of diverse structure. Hans argued persuasively that we should not lose track of the second possibility. Three years later, our studies and those of others suggest that proposition 2 is most likely. Hans' view was that anticancer drugs are largely plant products that enter the body through the digestive tract. Hence, the system may have a long phyllogenetic existence. I remember his joy when he learned that we had identified the system in the proximal tubular cell of the dogfish shark!

The editors of this volume instructed authors that the text should stick to specific experiences of importance. For me and my family, knowing Hans as friend and colleague was a rare opportunity. During Hans' and Lina's last visit with us in Boston, a remarkable event occurred. Hans didn't work for a whole day and night! Instead, we talked, drank wine, ate, listened to music, and shared experiences and friendship—all day. No, he wasn't sick. There was a major hurricane outside and we were housebound! I suspect that this was the only day in his life that he didn't work, read, or otherwise expand his horizons and help us all in the process—but it took a hurricane!

Hans was a friend and an inspiration. It is one of my life's greatest pleasures to have been one of his many students, colleagues, and friends.

3

Leonardo Bianchi, Basel

"SHOULD WE INVITE HIM?"
Hans Popper and the Basel Liver Weeks

BASEL, OCTOBER 16, 1989   The symposium, "Proteins in the Regulation of Hepatic Genes," was running. A rather dull discussion following
a presentation on transforming growth factors was suddenly enlivened by
a stimulating comment from far away in the rear of the lecture theatre. I
stirred, with a strange feeling of déjà vu—Hans was with us again, sparkling with scientific curiosity and bright ideas. I looked around—but alas
there was no Hans. I lapsed into reverie and became absorbed as I remembered how it all began.

FREIBURG (WEST GERMANY) 1965   I was working in my office in Surgical
Pathology in the Ludwig Aschoff House, the Pathology Department of the
University of Freiburg. One morning, the door opened and an impulsive
man, short of stature, came in and shook hands: "I am Hans Popper, may I
visit you?" I was startled. Convinced that he had missed the right door, I
offered to introduce him to the head of the department. "No, it is not your
boss I want to see. It is from the young people I can learn and I would prefer
to look at slides with you! What are you working on?" Still hesitating, I
pointed vaguely to my daily pile of liver and spleen biopsies. The next hour
or two was an unforgettable lesson for me—Hans Popper sitting at my microscope reading liver biopsies while I attempted to present the clinical aspects. He suddenly interrupted me: ". . . Don't tell me what clinicians are
writing down—I will tell you from the biopsy what is wrong with the pa-

13

tient." And since then this has become my credo in reading biopsies. From a case of cholestasis Hans detected a Sirius red-stained section—a preparation with which he obviously was not familiar. He got excited about the brilliant demonstration of bilirubin and the sensitivity of the stain for collagen. He quickly pulled out his famous notebook from his pocket to write down the details of the method. In return he encouraged me to "make a diastase-PAS, you will have much fun!"

THE FIRST INTERNATIONAL CONGRESS OF LIVER DISEASES IN FREIBURG, 1967   Two years later, in October 1967, I met Hans Popper again in Freiburg. Ludwig Heilmeyer was chairman of the First International Congress on Liver Diseases. "Jaundice" was the major topic, and Hans Popper was on the program as moderator of one of the sessions. He presented a paper on drug-induced jaundice. I had finished my thesis on liver biopsy diagnosis and differential diagnosis in hepatitis. At the welcome party, Heilmeyer wanted to introduce me to Hans Popper and to discuss my work. Popper immediately recognized me—his memory was legendary—and he led me to a quiet corner where for a long time we "talked shop" on liver histology. I left the party late but with an invitation to contribute a chapter to the forthcoming volume of *Progress in Liver Diseases*.

At this same meeting, Herbert Falk had invited the group to a farewell dinner-dance at Bad Krozingen, a spa some 15 miles from Freiburg. The party guests traveled by bus. There was uproarious festivity until late in the night. Hans and Lina Popper, however, were scheduled for an early morning flight from Basel and wished to leave for their hotel in Freiburg before the party was over. My wife Emmeli offered to drive them in our car; the only problem was that we had our Airedale terrier, Vivo, in the car. Hans claimed to like dogs and indicated that he would feel quite comfortable sitting beside our dog. Fenton Schaffner also wanted to join us. When we got to the car, Lina took the front seat and Fenton and Hans slipped into the back. Then Win Arias appeared, also wishing a lift back to Freiburg. Emmeli appeared embarrassed, but Hans generously invited him to get in. Three gentlemen and one dog in the rear of an old Volvo! Hans, squeezed between Fenton and the dog, appeared somewhat concerned about what was happening. When he realized that the dog was obedient and well behaved, he extended his hand and said to the dog: "Hello, you are a nice fellow—my name is Hans Popper."

The symposium "Icterus" was deemed such a great success that Herbert Falk agreed to sponsor a further meeting in 1970. This time the theme was "Alcohol and the Liver," and Hans Popper was chairman.

Influenced largely by Hans Popper, the third major Freiburg Liver Meeting in October 1973 was called "Drugs and the Liver." Rudi Schmid acted as chairman. Hans gave a splendid lecture, "Structural Aspects of Hepatic Biotransformation," at that time one of his favored hobbyhorses. A highlight in October 1973 was the 2-day premeeting, "Collagen Metabolism in the Liver," chaired by Hans. Here he was in his proper element: He considered fibrosis of the liver as the major factor for cirrhosis, morbidity, and death from liver disease, and he deeply deplored the limited understanding of the mechanisms involved in fibrogenesis and in the breakdown of collagen. For this premeeting it was his idea to bring together experts, on the one hand, in aspects of collagen and matrix research with no or only marginal interest in the liver and on the other hepatologists investigating fibrosis of the liver. From such an exchange of experience between basic scientists and hepatologists he expected what he liked to call "cross-fertilization"— the hepatologists would learn new methods and how to apply them to their specific hepatologic problems, and the basic scientists would be encouraged to use the liver as a model to answer their questions, this in turn leading to progress in liver research. The meeting attracted a large and enthusiastic audience. In a masterful "Overview of Past and Future of Hepatic Collagen Metabolism" at the end of the meeting, Hans defined the current state of the art and by posing questions stimulated many research groups to intensify their studies on liver fibrosis. A further outcome of this challenging meeting was the appearance of many publications and further international conferences on this topic.

Encouraged by this success, Hans repeated the experiment a year later with the "cross-fertilizing" conference, "Pathogenesis and Mechanisms of Liver Cell Necrosis." Again, the concept of this type of scientific encounter or congress met with great enthusiasm.

Hans then thought it useful to combine one or two such scientific meetings with the already traditional International Falk Liver Congresses. Thanks to his continuing initiative and the generous sponsorship of Herbert Falk, these Falk Conferences became established (see Fig. 1 in photo section).

BASEL LIVER WEEKS   I was privileged to act as the organizing secretary for these events and this, indeed, became one of the most rewarding experiences of my life. I was permitted to assist actively in the planning and preparations of meetings and witnessed that marvelous and unique facility that enabled Hans to correctly anticipate issues and topics that would become important. He planned a meeting 2 years ahead so that precisely at the time the meeting took place the topic was making a significant impact on hepatology.

The main congress in 1976 was entitled "Liver and Bile" (Chairman: Fenton Schaffner). For the satellite conference, Hans planned a fascinating program, "Membrane Alterations as Basis of Liver Injury," to "bring approach, information and technology in the rapidly expanding field of cell membranes together and to apply it not only to the biology of the liver but, more importantly, to the understanding, diagnosis and eventual therapy of liver diseases" (Hans Popper in his introduction to the meeting).

To plan and to draw up a program with Hans was a most interesting and exciting experience. An outline program of topics for the half-day sessions was drafted and candidate moderators were discussed. Although the speakers for the "Membrane" meeting (as for all the satellite conferences) were supposed to be mainly basic scientists, Hans was anxious to engage moderators with a particular hepatic interest in order to make the sessions more "liverish." However, he also took care to maintain a balance between European and overseas participants, so as not to overstretch the generous financial support by Herbert Falk.

By the time the organizers met to discuss the program for the main symposium, the outline for the premeeting was already more or less determined. Membrane alterations are also crucial in the mechanism of cholestasis, and this established a close link between the premeeting and the main symposium. The advantage of this was that Hans succeeded in attracting scientists active in membrane research, who, in addition, could be secured as speakers for the main congress, although they would have been hard to get for a postgraduate liver meeting. These basic lectures did, indeed, give the main congress a special flavor.

The deadline for inviting the speakers was set at 1 year prior to the meeting. But it is far from the mark if the reader assumes that by then no more changes in the program were made. Whenever Hans was at a meeting anywhere in the world and read or got to hear of new and exciting results he would immediately try to engage the respective scientist and to integrate his talk in our program.

Hans disliked unorganized presentations. He got uneasy about speakers who talked too long at the meeting, but he wanted to be correct. After a full lecture day, Hans enjoyed the comments given by faculty members; it happened that such comments stimulated him to develop new ideas that he would introduce into the next day's discussions (see Fig. 2 in photo section).

The best times to work on the Basel Liver Week programs were during Hans' trips to Europe. I remember picking him up with Lina at Zurich Airport in May 1978. During the 1-hour drive to Basel I got a perfect summary of a meeting in Atlantic City from which he had just come. In addition, he made suggestions as to what would be of interest for inclusion in our program.

In the pleasant surroundings of a Black Forest inn—Herbert Falk had invited us for a dinner at the Weserei in Kandern—we discussed the pre-meeting to be held in October 1979. We wanted this topic to be related to and follow up on the previous "Membrane" meeting. Hans already had quite clear concepts. While the previous meeting dealt with well-defined structural entities—the cell membranes—the focus should now be on mechanisms, interactions of cells, and transmission of signals from, to, and within liver cells. But we had to find a "catchy" title. Everybody at the table, while enjoying a delicious dessert, made suggestions: "How liver cells talk to each other?" Hans turned up his nose. "Social behavior of liver cells?" Hans grumbled. "Communication of liver cells?" Hans had a broad grin, pointed an approving finger at the proposer, and leapt to his feet. "That's it!" he exclaimed.

The discussions went on during the annual workshop of our Liver Study Group, which in May 1978 was in Zurich. Selection and exclusion of topics this time were particularly difficult; to bring the abstract term "communication" into context with the liver and its diseases was merely a matter of preference. The menu cards at lunch and dinner proved too small for our outlines and lists of contributors; we escaped to the lecture room to continue on the blackboard (Fig. 3). While we discussed back and forth, Hans always made me feel that *I* was the head of the Basel Liver Week.

The main symposium was supposed to be called "Virus and the Liver" (Dame Sheila Sherlock had agreed to chair it). It seemed reasonable, therefore, to include in the premeeting some discussion of the immunological interactions in the liver. Hans agreed—but his face was a picture-book, indicating that he was not particularly enthusiastic about this. Indeed, with a disdainful gesture, he confessed that he felt confused about the profusion of data on immunological reactions and that he did not believe in their relevance in liver diseases. "Nevertheless, we need an immunology session," he confirmed, "but I will not give a summary!" We decided to ask somebody else to review the immunological part and to present an overview of it in the framework of the "Virus and Liver" congress.

In order to extend the Liver Week to a full week, Herbert Falk wanted us to consider an additional 1-day session. Hans proposed a histopathology seminar; he enthusiastically bubbled over with ideas on how to organize it and whom to invite. When we disagreed on a candidate participant, he tried to persuade me: "You are right, he has no fire, but . . . be smart, invite him, that will not do you any harm. . . ." With a twinkle in his eyes he said, "perhaps you will be invited to his place in return . . . it is a lovely town!" I made Hans consider the enormous organizational work that a slide seminar required. With a malicious smile, he tempted me: "Look, it is a challenge . . . and I have something quite new in histology: . . . an H + E slide and my brain." Who could have resisted?

The premeetings of the next two Basel Liver Weeks continued the general theme of the previous topics: "Structural Carbohydrates in the Liver" in 1982 and "Modulation of Liver Cell Expression" in 1986. Again, the intention was to bring together investigators from diverse nonhepatologic disciplines who ordinarily would have little contact with one another, and, again, Hans could cajole all those people he wanted and convince them of the wisdom of coming to Basel. These get-togethers were appreciated by both basic scientists and hepatologists. Highlights of these satellite meetings were undoubtedly the summaries Hans presented at the end of the meeting. What the audience savored like a delicious postprandial liqueur was the result of hard work: Hans missed not 1 minute of the 2 days' lectures, filling a whole notebook with his remarks; in the intermissions he contacted speakers to clarify with them whatever he felt he had not fully understood. When everybody else went to bed after the famous Falk dinner parties, Hans got to work again; or else he got up very early in the morning, did his Canadian Air Force exercises and worked on his summary. At breakfast or even after lunch on the last day, he would hand over to me carefully edited handwritten notes; he was lucky in that I was always able to keep my promise and to have "lantern slides" ready in time for his scheduled summary presentations. Hans worked incredibly hard during these meetings. And yet, when those of us who were much younger were exhausted, he continued to be excellent company; there was always fun and laughter at the Poppers' table at the dinner parties.

What is the future of the Basel Liver Weeks—if there are any—without Hans? He left us a rich heritage, and he was a genius who taught us many lessons. We can only aspire to follow in his footsteps.

4

Baruch S. Blumberg, Philadelphia

THE HEPATITIS RESEARCH GROUP
Institute for Cancer Research
Fox Chase Cancer Center

Hans Popper had a dramatic style and, often, a profound effect on scientists and friends with whom he came into contact. We, that is, those of us at the Clinical Research Division at the Institute for Cancer Research of the Fox Chase Cancer Center in Philadelphia, were no exception. I would like to recall several episodes to illustrate the important influence Hans had on our group.

None of us had been involved in the hepatitis field or studies on the liver until, in 1964, we found a protein-containing substance in the blood of an Australian aborigine that we later showed to be the surface antigen of a hepatitis virus. However, our initial findings were viewed with considerable skepticism by the established workers in the field, a group we collectively referred to as the "hepatitis cats." Their disbelief was by no means unwarranted. There had been many candidate hepatitis viruses, and the approach we had used was unconventional. In addition, we were essentially unknown in the field.

In 1968, we were invited to present our data to the Hepatitis Board of the U.S. Army. The Board included many members of the hepatitis establishment, including Hans Popper, who had long enjoyed a distinguished position because of his early prominence in the field. Our reception was by no means hostile, but certainly very critical with the message that further evidence, to be produced by ourselves and others, would be required in order for our claims to gain acceptance. (There were also other obstacles; for example, one of our papers had been rejected by the *Annals of Internal Medicine*, which thought our presumption was too great.) Some time after the meeting, Hans came to speak to us. This was probably the first time I had met him, with the possible exception of having heard him lecture, when I was a student at the College of Physicians and Surgeons, at The Mount Sinai Hospital (Hans' institution), which had an academic connection with our school.

Hans was extremely encouraging. He accepted our data and arguments and encouraged us to continue our research diligently; in effect, we received his support. In later discussions within our group, we often recalled how important this was to us at a period when we needed a sympathetic ear among those who would have a major role in evaluating our claims.

This was not the only occasion in which Hans' academic interest was crucial. By 1971, we had already introduced the method to produce hepatitis B vaccine. It was difficult, initially, to generate any interest in it and when we did it was often critical, since the process we had used was novel, that is, producing a vaccine from the blood of hepatitis B carriers. Hans, on the other hand, was all optimism when we spoke with him. As always, he was prepared to accept new possibilities, and his support encouraged us to find a commercial collaborator who could, and did, develop our ideas.

My colleague, Anna O'Connell, knew Hans for about as long as I. When I told her that I had been invited to write this remembrance, she spontaneously said, "Hans Popper was, to me, pure delight. He enjoyed science and wasn't as serious as most pathologists." She went on to say that for any given situation he could relate to a previous event, tragic or happy, and enrich the present problem with his considerable and easily accessed experience. She concluded by adding that even at boring meetings, "you could have a good time with Hans."

Tom London, who had also known Hans for many years, recalled that, even into his 80s, Hans would attend scientific meetings and provide the final summations. Further, he didn't fall asleep toward the end of the sessions as even younger, but less hardy, scientists would frequently do. Whenever we went to his laboratory, he would ask us, "Where are the slides?" It was the data and the visual image of health and disease under the all-revealing microscope that drove Hans' intellectual machine.

Perhaps my most vivid recollection of Hans was during the Basel Liver Week in Freiburg in 1973 (see Fig. 4 in photo section). Hans appeared to be everywhere, discussing the scientific papers, leading people to dinner, initiating the dancing sessions, singing songs. He was bright, quick-stepped, effusive, positive, enjoying with enthusiasm those meetings that, in a strange way, seemed to revolve around his personality. The photographs taken on that occasion bring back to me, and I hope to others, the happy memories all of us will retain of a wonderful friend and a scientist who gave structure and content to the field of medical research that he embraced and nurtured.

Acknowledgment: This work was supported by USPHS grants CA-40737, RR-05895, and CA-06927 from the National Institutes of Health and by an appropriation from the Commonwealth of Pennsylvania.

5

James L. Boyer, New Haven

Three things stand out most in my mind about Hans Popper: first, his enormous intellect and memory, which never seemed to flag despite his advancing years; second, his devotion to the liver and the science of hepatology in all of its widest ramifications; and third and most important, the unbounding enthusiasm with which he greeted whatever activity he found himself involved in.

I first came to know Hans personally when I was appointed to the Council of the American Association for the Study of Liver Diseases (AASLD) in 1975–1976. As the founder of this society, Hans served as honorary councillor and remained throughout a guiding influence. Although the Association was now guided by its officers, and Hans was extremely careful not to interfere with the ideas of others, it was amazing how often the group would be locked in debate, often late in the evening, when Hans, having just raised his head from what seemed like deep slumber, would make a brief remark or observation that inevitably had the effect of swaying the entire group. He almost always was the fairest in evaluating the merits of others, and he usually favored younger, less well-known individuals when such a choice would help promote their careers. Indeed, he had an unusual ability to make so many people feel that they were quite special and important.

It was this latter characteristic that had such an influence on my own relationship with Hans and that came quite unexpectedly, since I had grown up in the Klatskin crowd, and, for reasons that probably had more to due with style than substance, I had been slow to appreciate Hans' special talents.

Shortly after becoming an AASLD council member, I learned that Hans was the one who could always be counted on to provide new ideas, information, and insight. As the years went by, I found myself looking forward to these meetings, particularly because I knew that Hans would always have something engaging to discuss that was unrelated to the meeting and that would set me thinking in new ways. Often this related to common research interests or to new discoveries in some aspect of hepatology. His well-known ability to keep up with all of the hepatologic literature during these last years was remarkable. He was probably the only person capable of summarizing the field. He was also fun to be with because of his infectious enthusiasm. What a treat to sit next to him on a plane trip or bus ride during a social outing at an international meeting! And, if Lina were there, you had an added bonus. Discussions ranged from politics to science, from their days in Vienna to tales of life in the American army. I remember well a special afternoon between the EASL and the IASL meetings in Berne, Switzerland in 1984. It was a lovely day, and Hans wanted to take a train ride to Grindlewald, high in the Alps. He had not been there for years and reminisced about his youth when he and his family used to come for vacations before the war. I remember little of the conversation, other than that it was wide-ranging as usual. I simply remember how pleasant it was to have this unique opportunity to share this afternoon with Hans even though I sensed he knew it was to be his last visit there.

Hans was always learning as he was teaching. He took a keen interest over the years in our research as he did with the research of many. Even a brief phone conversation would never end without some exchange of information. Often, a new idea or concept would appear in one of his timely summaries of a meeting or overview. His interest in us was enormously important, as it was a source of inspiration and stimulus to renew the effort.

When it came to planning a meeting or a conference, Hans could always be counted on to provide information on just who would be best to report the newest information on a given topic. He was seldom wrong.

I cannot say that there was any one particular aspect of my career or professional work that Hans specifically influenced. His impact was much broader. There is no doubt that he was influential in my becoming a council member of the AASLD at a relatively young age. His recommendations helped in my receiving invitations to participate in Falk Symposia, particularly when I was asked to serve as president in 1986 of the Basel Liver Week. He thought a lot about the leadership of hepatology and was influential in my election to the council and presidency of IASL. He was particularly interested in our work on mechanisms of bile secretion and cholestasis. I remember one occasion when I spoke at a meeting in New York on cholestasis emphasizing the role of the paracellular pathway and concluded by showing a drawing that Arnold Rich had published in 1925 in his monograph on jaundice (1), to emphasize that this concept was not new. Hans came up to me immediately afterward at the break and enlightened me to the fact that Rich had spent a sabbatical in Vienna and had learned this concept from Eppinger. Subsequently, I was informed in a letter from the Rumanian hepatologist, I. Pavel, that Eppinger had learned this from him (2). Whenever I spoke on the subject of cholestasis, Hans would ask how I explained the well-known pathologic finding of canalicular dilatation, since to his mind this implied that pressure should be increased in the canalicular space, and yet it seemed likely that the pressures should be equalized as the junctional barriers were disrupted. His question remains to be answered but may have more to do with alterations in membrane turnover during cholestatic liver injury, which leads to an imbalance between insertion and recovery (exocytosis versus endocytosis) of the apical canalicular membrane surface.

Hans also imparted to me, as he did to others, a sense of striving that, for himself, he likened to a ". . . restless Faustian drive" (3). This striving for new knowledge continued unabated until the end of his life. Hans Popper believed passionately in international communication and was the undisputed father of international hepatology. He did not particularly like to dwell on the past, telling me once when I suggested he write a history of the development of the field of hepatology [he, writing and working, subsequently did (4)] that he much preferred to spend his time thinking about the future. So should we.

References

1. Rich A. The pathogenesis of the forms of jaundice. *Bull Johns Hopkins Hosp* 1930; 47:338–77.
2. Pavel I. La cholestase intrahepatique. *Sem Hop Paris* 1975; 51:1195–8.
3. Popper H. Vienna and the liver. In: Brunner H, Thaler H, eds. *Hepatology: a festschrift for Hans Popper*. New York: Raven Press, 1985:13.
4. Popper H. History of the American Association for the Study of Liver Diseases. *Hepatology* 1982; 2:874–8.

6

Thomas C. Chalmers, Boston

I believe that I first met Hans Popper when we both attended the first CIBA conference on liver disease, organized and run in London by Sheila Sherlock in 1950. It was attended by an exciting group of relatively young people whose research interests were confined to the liver. I don't remember whether or not Hans was the consummate meeting attender that he evolved into, but I am sure he had a lot to say about many of the presentations. I was there because in the 3 years after my residency I had been doing a fair amount of clinical research on patients with alcoholic liver disease at the Boston City Hospital under the tutelage of Charles Davidson, and for some reason he was unable to attend the meeting.

Three years later, I attended my first meeting of the American Association for the Study of the Liver at the Hektoen Institute of the Cook County Hospital in Chicago. The Association was just 4 or 5 years old, and there was already a formal structure of officers, but I do clearly remember that Hans ran the meeting. Five years later, I succeeded Wade Volweiler as president of the Association, but my best memories of that period were that Hans really ran the organization through the then-permanent secretary Fenton Schaffner and the annually elected president. In my year as president, we had a special meeting at the World Congress of Gastroenterology in Washington, D.C., in the spring of 1958, and Hans, Fenton, and Sheila Sherlock organized and started the International Association for the Study of the Liver, which is now an equally flourishing organization. We had another exciting aspect of my year as president in that Stan Harttroft and a few other members of the board fought vigorously to start a new journal to be called *Liver*, pushed by Henry Stratton, who had started the journal *Blood* and dreamed of an equally successful liver journal. I was strenuously opposed to the proliferation of specialty journals and thought that the journal *Gastroenterology* should be the forum for the publication of articles on hepatology. Hans illustrated one of his most able characteristics, that of mediator and fence-straddler, suppressing his strong desire to edit such a new journal, because he did not want to see the field splintered by opposing ideas. As it turned out, I couldn't have been more wrong, and there are now any number of liver journals, with no deterioration at all in the quality of *Gastroenterology*. That was an eventful year for me because I was able to see first-hand how a bright, able, and forward-thinking man could achieve what was needed by patience and forbearance in diplomatic dealings with all factions. It was a harbinger of his success in pulling together the Mount Sinai staff and trustees into the start of a great medical school.

Those days were the heyday of liver function tests, and Hans was undoubtedly the world leader in trying to explain the biochemical changes in morphological terms. Most of the clinical observational research was hampered by a lack of scientific rigor, and I don't think at that time Hans had begun the practice of interpreting all slides without knowledge of the clinical data. However, sometime around then, he began to appreciate the importance of controlling bias by reading slides without hints as to what he should find, and he maintained this discipline as long as he worked. It is pathetic how few morphologists follow his teachings in their clinical service or research activities.

I saw a first-hand example of his enormous ability to discern changes in the morphology of the liver under the light microscope when we, many years later, collaborated on a paper concerned with the morphology of chronic hepatitis. Hans had organized a group of worldwide hepatologists to meet for a consensus conference on the morphological distinctions between the more benign chronic persistent hepatitis and the more serious chronic active hepatitis. The group, known affectionately as the "gnomes of Zurich," came up with a distinction that has been followed with various modifications ever since. Years later, when I was at Mount Sinai and searching around for research that an academic medical center administrator could perform, I persuaded a medical student, Eve Kirschner, now a hepatologist on the west coast, to carry out a follow-up study of patients Fenton Schaffner had biopsied 10 or more years before to document the predictability of the lesions. I had a warm spot in my heart for Dr. Kirschner because she became interested in hepatology in medical school for the same reason that I did, namely that she had a serum bilirubin around 3 or 4 and we were both classic examples of Gilbert's syndrome. We resurrected the liver biopsies obtained by Fenton and had them reread by three pathologists, with the request that they stick their necks out as to whether they were examples of chronic active or chronic persistent hepatitis. Each pathologist read the slides under different codes on two occasions, 6 months apart. Hans led the three in the reproducibility of his opinions; he was remarkably consistent. Unfortunately, the number of patients was far too small to give reliable data on the predictability, but we all learned something about the Type II error from that experience. And I became immensely impressed that when someone like Hans was reading the biopsies the reports are amazingly reproducible.

During the early years of my acquaintance with Hans, I attended meetings of a fascinating hepatologically inclined group, the Subcommittee on the Liver of the Armed Forces Epidemiological Board. It was originally chaired by Cecil Watson of the University of Minnesota and subsequently by Charles Davidson and Hans Popper. There may have been others after I stopped going to the meetings. This committee was set up by the U.S. Army to advise how money appropriated for hepatology research, primarily hepatitis, should be spent. But the meetings turned out to be marvelous colloquia at which the members presented their recent research for discussion by each other. It was an ideal milieu in which to make decisions about how future research should be funded. Hans was an outspoken and vigorous contributor to the meetings, respected by everyone.

This might be the time to comment further on Popper's contributions to the intellectual ferment and value of all the meetings he attended, beginning with the CIBA symposium and the Macy conferences and the Subcommittee on the Liver, and extending to the more formal annual meetings of the Liver Association and the Falk Symposia held every fall for the last few years. Their natural history illustrates a sort of intellectual senescence, which seems to be as inevitable as biological aging, and against which Popper fought, albeit possibly not as successfully as he did his own biological aging. The small group meetings to which everybody came, anxious to learn from each other and argue with each other, were obviously the most productive and successful to my mind. As each organization grew older, there became a need to bring in more people and make the deliberations available by publication for those who did not attend. This process eliminated the informal presentation of research in progress and soon each of the surviving organizations became a formal medical society with published abstracts. People boast about the fact that the liver associations Hans founded have grown to have more than 2,000 attendees at a meeting. How successful, how pitiful! The opportunity for spontaneity, for tossing around wild ideas, has been lost.

Hans did his bit to oppose this trend toward lesser productivity in several ways. First, he became a consummate attender of the meetings in the sense that he paid intense attention to everything that was said and distinguished himself as a synthesizer and commentator extraordinaire. With exaggerated modesty he would reintroduce into these large convocations as if they were small ones the kind of stimulating thoughts that occurred to him and that everyone else would have liked to have thought.

Hans was also highly successful in making the most of the social aspects of those meetings. It is of interest that we hepatologists drank a lot at the end of a long day of heavy thinking and listening, and the alcohol removed some of the inhibitions imposed by the formality of the larger meetings. Hans could be especially sharp and perceptive after three vodka martinis, from which he omitted the vermouth. He drank only vodka because of an unscientific but attractive belief that it might be the congeners in alcohol that injured the liver and that the more pure the alcohol the more one could drink without damage.

After I succeeded him as the head of Mount Sinai, I achieved great pleasure and satisfaction by dropping in on him around 6 p.m. for an hour or two of conversation stimulated by his drinking vodka and me drinking gin. My reason for dropping by was my need to unburden myself of my worst administrative problems, but we actually ended up talking much more about our research.

It might be of interest to recount how I happened to succeed Hans as president of The Mount Sinai Medical Center and dean of the medical school. During the 2 years between Hans' retirement as chairman of pathology and my arriving at Mount Sinai, the search committee, of which he was the leading light while also serving as president and dean, went through a list of 200 potential names looking for a successor to George James, the first president and dean. My name was not on the list. During those 2 years, I was at the clinical center of NIH and served on the committee to choose Fogarty scholars, who would be supported for up to 6 months of residence at NIH with participation in whatever intellectual activity at the institution they thought appropriate. Anxious to have a few hepatologists around, I had recruited Cecil Watson and Charles Davidson, but Hans Popper could not accept our proffered appointment because he was too busy at Mount Sinai. Finally, at a meeting of the American Gastroenterological Association in late May 1973 in New Orleans, I told him that we were going to have to fill the slot with someone else and could not keep it open for him any longer. He said he would have to decline again because they had been unable to find anyone to succeed him at Sinai and he could not leave until they did. On the spur of the moment he asked me if I would be interested in the job. I said I might, because the second Nixon administration had replaced the man who had hired me at NIH, Bob Marston. I had supper with a small group of the selection committee in New York in mid-June, returned a week later, and after that meeting Hans told me that he thought he could arrange a unanimous vote for me by the committee. I accepted the job early in July, and, on October 1, I started at Mount Sinai and Hans started a long relationship with NIH. I do believe that his persuasiveness had a lot to do with the rapidity of the institution's making an offer and with my accepting it so promptly.

I hope and expect that someone else contributing to this memorial to Hans will describe his tremendously productive contributions to the clinical and basic research going on at NIH. I get a great deal of satisfaction out of the realization that I brought him there.

The Mount Sinai School of Medicine is a great institution, which will be even greater in the future, and there is no doubt in my mind that Hans Popper is its father and founder. He may have come to Mount Sinai Hospital in 1957 with no greater ambition than to succeed the famous Paul Klemperer as chairman of the Department of Pathology. However, I suspect that the idea of a medical school began to germinate in his fertile mind not long after his arrival. He gave three reasons why the hospital should eventually start a school of medicine. First, the pre- and early postwar period, when the brightest Jewish graduates of American medical schools could not get posts for house staff training at the famous hospitals, such as Massachusetts General or Presbyterian, greatly benefitted Mount Sinai, because it could easily recruit some of the brightest graduates around. When the best hospitals in the country overcame this disgraceful prejudice, Mount Sinai suffered because it could not compete without a school of its own. Second, the hospital had become both famous and excellent because of its clinically related research; it needed basic science departments to maintain that leadership. Third, there was a recognized national need for more medical school graduates.

Hans was way ahead of his time in recognizing that the days of the traditional basic science departments in an academic medical center were numbered. The explosion of techniques for understanding molecular biology and related disciplines was wiping out the distinctions among the basic science departments. The biochemists were thinking in physiologic terms and vice versa. Hans tried to start a medical school with basic scientists doing their research and teaching in noncompartmentalized biology. He failed because the idea was too revolutionary to attract really good people. In the clinical sphere, he felt that he did not have to worry about the quality of patient care and teaching because of the superb abilities of the clinical staff of the hospital, so he took a bold step, choosing Dr. Solomon Berson, a scientist with minimal clinical training, as the first chairman of medicine after the start of the school. Had Berson not died suddenly barely 2 years after taking the job, he would have been the first chairman of a department of medicine to win the Nobel Prize, which was awarded to his coworker Roslyn Yalow several years after his death. Hans also showed his perception of what was going to be important in the next few years by choosing as the first president and dean of the medical school a public-health-oriented man, Dr. George James, and by building the largest and most successful department of community medicine in the country, headed by Dr. Kurt Deuschle.

As in the case of Case Western Reserve Medical School, many of the innovative methods of teaching adapted by Mount Sinai's school have not survived the rigorous pressures of financial and faculty overwork problems, but the nidus started by Hans continued to have influence in slowing the academic regression toward the mean (mediocre). Innovations in medical education are truly hard to bring about!

My job at Mount Sinai for 10 years was made much easier by the fact that Hans had established with the old guard of the hospital and with the trustees the realization that the best patient care is found in institutions that attract the best people as undergraduate students, graduates in training, and young faculty, and that a scientifically rigorous environment is the best way to accomplish that job. He and I both truly believed that good science is the primary ingredient of good patient care.

This memory of Hans is nowhere near as eloquent as that published by Rudi Schmid and Steven Schenker in *Hepatology*, the official organ of the American Association for the Study of Liver Diseases, but the enthusiasm for him as a person and as a scientist is the same. Although I never collaborated to any great degree in research with Hans Popper, I owe him a tremendous debt of gratitude in teaching me how to function in medical organizations and for laying the groundwork for my having had the best 10 years of my life at Mount Sinai.

7

Whan Kook Chung, Seoul

CHRONIC HEPATITIS B IN KOREA

I first met Dr. Hans Popper in 1961 when I was engaged in a study of viral hepatitis in the Korean Army Medical Corps, which was still struggling for postwar recovery. For more than 25 years after that fortunate encounter, Dr. Popper was my teacher and mentor and exerted inestimable influence on me both professionally and personally, constantly providing me with timely encouragement and useful advice.

One day toward the end of 1960, Col. Irey (chief of the medical division of the Eighth U.S. Army) and I were examining tissue slides I had prepared of arsenical hepatitis cases. Because we were puzzled by some of them, Col. Irey proposed that we show the slides to Dr. Popper, who was to come to Seoul in June of the following year as consultant to the United States Army. I was delighted that Col. Irey, at my suggestion, promised to make arrangements for Dr. Popper to deliver lectures and conduct a case discussion at the ROK Capital Army Hospital when he came to Seoul. This is how my association with Dr. Popper began.

During and after the Korean War, while in the Korean Army Medical Corps, I noted severe morbidity among Korean soldiers, often resulting in mortality, without clear reasons. They did not exhibit jaundice, but I performed hepatic tests. When I observed abnormal results, I performed liver biopsies on them. Complex and time-consuming follow-up studies were carried out on these patients under difficult conditions typical of the postwar period. At that time, the etiology of viral hepatitis was shrouded in mystery, and theories, if any, were based on speculation.

When I met Dr. Popper, there were two questions I wanted to ask him. Was there any relationship between acute icteric viral hepatitis, which was prevalent in Korea, and chronic hepatic disease? What was his opinion on the histologic entity of anicteric asymptomatic hepatitis, which, as described below, was then prevalent among the recruits of the ROK Army?

When I was working at the RTC in Nonsan just after the Korean War, I felt that it would be possible to detect a large number of patients with anicteric asymptomatic hepatitis among the recruits by a screening survey with serum transaminases. An actual survey was carried out in February 1961, just before Dr. Popper came to Seoul, in collaboration with Capt. Alfred M. Prince from the 406 MGL of the United States Army in Japan. He subsequently discovered serum hepatitis antigen in our biopsy material obtained from anicteric hepatitis cases. Of 1,906 recruits surveyed, about 80 were found to have repeatedly abnormal transaminases. Thirty-two of them were hospitalized and biopsied two to three times during a 3-month period of hospitalization.

We conducted an intensive study on the 32 hospitalized subjects, including weekly determination by the then-available liver function tests. The findings were amazingly interesting: the 32 army recruits were clinically well and active, yet their liver function was in most cases chronically abnormal or fluctuating between normality and abnormality. Similarly, liver biopsies showed chronic hepatitis with no trend toward improvement even in those subjects in whom liver function seemed to get normalized. What was more striking was that serial liver biopsies showed development of cirrhosis in four of the subjects.

Finally, with the help of Col. Irey and Capt. Prince, I was able to meet Dr. Popper in June 1961 at the Capital Army Hospital, to which I was assigned at that time, and he gave a lecture there.

In order to facilitate Dr. Popper's understanding and to hear his opinion, I assembled in a ward eight patients who were suspected to fall into the above-mentioned two categories. At the foot of each bed was placed a microscope with slides from serial biopsies, which in most cases spanned many years. On the wall over each bed was shown a summary of the clinical and laboratory data. Dr. Popper was deeply impressed and told Capt. Prince later that he had never seen such an in-depth study in the United States or Europe.

Next day, he flew with me to Taejon and visited the 63rd ROK Army Hospital, where he gave a lecture (see Fig. 5 in photo section). We had more discussions on anicteric hepatitis.

I presume this encounter led to his better understanding of me and Korean medicine, especially the picture of chronic hepatitis in Korea, and perhaps spurred him on to help me in further studies, to analyze these valuable materials, and to introduce them to the international medical world. Anyway, he invited me to come to his institution for research, which I gladly accepted. Thus, it was possible for me to study for 2 years (1962–1964) at The Mount Sinai Hospital, where my observations were consolidated under his guidance. During that time, Dr. Popper fully confirmed these observations. As a matter of fact, our cooperation resulted in one of the first descriptions of chronic hepatitis. This disease entity gradually became recognized at that time due to the availability of my liver biopsies and of serum transaminase activity determinations.

Sera from 9 of the 32 cases with anicteric hepatitis were available for HBsAg tests later, and 8 of them had HBsAg. The results emphasized the significance of the hepatitis B virus carrier state in the etiology of chronic hepatitis in Korea.

In retrospect, without Dr. Popper's help, my achievements in the world of medicine would have been buried permanently in oblivion.

Our knowledge of the natural history of chronic hepatitis was rather limited because few sequential studies including biopsies were available. For technical reasons, relatively few sequential biopsy studies of chronic viral hepatitis B were available; the initial acute hepatitis B was barely documented, since biopsies were then rarely performed in the acute stage of hepatitis. Moreover, most published sequential studies were complicated by therapeutic intervention.

After my return to Korea and to civilian life, I had an opportunity to conduct a long-term follow-up study of many patients with acute and chronic hepatitis B by means of liver biopsy. Many of these patients had had no exposure to hepatoxic drugs, alcohol abuse, or steroid therapy. Thus, I have been able to observe and study the natural evolution of chronic hepatitis B prevalent in Korea longer and in greater detail than anyone else. During the next 25 years, I visited Dr. Popper's laboratory frequently and obtained a great deal of advice from him about the pattern of progression of chronic hepatitis B. He always gave me kind and clear comments, and his instruction was immeasurably helpful in establishing the natural history of this disease.

After histological evaluation of my serial biopsies of patients with chronic hepatitis B in Korea and examination of liver biopsy materials from patients treated with antiviral agents by the Stanford group in the United States, he began to doubt the validity of the then current emphasis on the transformation of chronic active hepatitis into cirrhosis resulting from continuous progression of periportal necroinflammation (piecemeal necrosis) and the disappearance of the lobular architecture. Thereafter, his emphasis was placed on episodes of acute exacerbation of lobular necroinflammation in the evolution of chronic hepatitis B. He suggested that in chronic active hepatitis B in Korea, such episodes were reflected as a cluster of hepatocytes in acinar arrangement replacing the circumscribed area of collapse (circumscribed hepatic necrosis).

My observation on circumscribed hepatic necrosis in Korea, which led him to reach the conclusion mentioned above, is outlined as follows: Thirty-five sequential biopsy specimens obtained from 14 Korean adult patients at intervals of 20 days to 11 years were studied and correlated with clinical findings. In 11 of them, a severe circumscribed alteration of the lobular parenchyma was noted, and, in three, similar lesions of a minor degree were found. The circumscribed hepatic necrosis showed an acinar arrangement of altered hepatocytes surrounded by increased connective tissue, progressing to collapse. The lesion frequently followed histologically documented acute viral hepatitis but was found in the presence of chronic active hepatitis and was also preceded by chronic lobular hepatitis, which differs from the emphasized circumscribed lesion in diffuse lobular development. The lesion was frequently associated with transition to cirrhosis. It might be a factor in this process. It was usually accompanied by clinical manifestations of hepatic failure, followed by the death of the patient during observation, but recovery was also observed.

After a thorough review of the results of this observation, Dr. Popper suggested that I carry out further investigation to clarify whether replication of viral DNA in circumscribed hepatic necrosis is depressed or elevated, whether immune reactivity has changed, whether superinfection can be established, whether the lesion is found only in hepatitis B and, finally, whether the infection of hepatitis B virus occurs early in life or late. His conclusive comment was that whatever the result of these studies, the observation presented suggested a major role of parenchymal changes in the evolution of chronic hepatitis B. In addition, he not only emphasized the importance of lesions of the lobular parenchyma in the classification and evaluation of chronic hepatitis but also the role of the lesions in the development of hepatocellular carcinoma.

From then on, whenever he explained the progression of chronic hepatitis B at international conferences, he emphasized the role of the lobular parenchymal lesion and introduced the observation of circumscribed hepatic necrosis in Korea, unfailingly mentioning my name. This was a great encouragement for me.

For the development of hepatology in Korea and the promotion of Korea's national prestige, he also initiated an international scientific committee and an international medical meeting. In 1961, soon after he returned to the United States from Korea, Dr. Popper organized the Liver Slide Exchange Committee under which were rallied Asian hepatologists including Prof. Mayake, Prof. Amano, Prof. Miyazi, all from Japan, and Prof. Hou from Hong Kong, and myself from Korea. The primary purpose of this committee was to encourage Asian hepatologists and to promote friendship among them.

In 1982, upon the exhortation of Dr. Popper, many world authorities in liver disease attended the Seoul International Liver Symposium. He also made an arrangement to have the Falk Foundation provide us with financial support. These efforts of his resulted in the success of the symposium, which was well attended with enthusiasm and promoted Korea's prestige in hepatology.

By helping quite a number of young doctors from my department train in various outstanding medical research institutes in the United States, Dr. Popper enabled us to continue the progress of the virology and molecular biology of viral hepatitis in Korea. We are continuing to cooperate in this respect with researchers in the United States, especially with scholars of the National Institutes of Health and The Mount Sinai School of Medicine. As a consequence, we have been able to create an efficient and well-organized clinical and laboratory research center of hepatology in Seoul.

In appreciation of his meritorious dedication to the development of medical science in Korea, the Catholic University Medical College in Seoul conferred on him an honorary degree of doctor of medical science in July 1978, (Figs. 6 and 7), and in February 1982, the Government of the Republic of Korea decorated him with the Order of Mugungwha, which is only given to persons whom the people of Korea respect most highly (Fig. 8).

Dr. Popper lived a meaningful life, and his contributions to hepatology in Korea will always remain with us. I sincerely appreciate the help he gave me with my study of liver disease over the more than 25 years of our association. I will long remember him as a true friend and teacher.

8

Harold O. Conn, New Haven

Three episodes among many pleasant interactions that occurred between us over a period of almost 35 years endeared Hans Popper to me.

The first took place immediately after the annual meeting of the AASLD in 1972, the year of my presidency. He warmly congratulated me and said that he thought it was the best meeting we had ever had. I basked for a decade in the glow of that compliment. Some years later, during a discussion of Hans' role as the cytoskeleton of the AASLD among a group of past presidents, we realized that he had taken the time to make some such comment to each of us. Indeed, each year the annual meetings got better and better as each new president engrafted something new in his own image to the program format.

The second episode took place about 5 years before he died. I had returned from a sabbatical during which I had been granted an automatic 1-year extension on my VA research grant. Unfortunately, in the interim, new chiefs of research at both national and local levels had been appointed, and the extension had not been implemented. I was told that I was eligible to apply for a new 5-year grant but that my funds would be interrupted for about 3 months, even if my proposal were funded. In effect, failure to extend the grant functioned as a rejection of my application. This deprived me of the built-in "turnaround time," i.e., the opportunity to submit an amended proposal without interruption of funding. This meant that several of my long-term laboratory workers would be terminated. I was informed that I could rehire them after a few months if my proposal were approved. It was unlikely that these well-trained individuals would still be available after a 3-month hiatus without pay. I complained that after 28 consecutive years of funding my program was to be unintentionally dismantled because of an oversight. Everyone I spoke to as I went up the chain of command was sympathetic but either was unwilling to protest or predicted rejection of their protests. Indeed, the predictions were correct. The chief of research in the VA central office rejected our requests for a delay. I was free to submit an application or not; the hiatus would be short if I did so successfully and permanent if I didn't. At this point I spoke to Dr. Popper, who listened to the bureaucratic nonsense and then wrote a short letter. In essence he wrote that I had consistently done good work in the past, and that now if I applied, I lost, and if I didn't, I lost. "This is a catch 22," he said. He suggested that the funding be continued only if the application was reviewed favorably. His suggestion was taken, and funding was continued until my application was subsequently approved. I learned later from a colleague in the VA central office that "Popper's impeccable Talmudic logic" was unchallengeable. As he did so often in medical, pathologic, and administrative impasses, he reduced the problem to its essential elements, and the solution quickly became apparent and achievable.

The third episode occurred at an organizational meeting of the Hepatologic Nomenclature Project in 1974. It was presided over by an administrator from the National Institutes of Health who was not a hepatologist and who did not know most of the members of the hepatic inner sanctum. As the meeting convened, about 35 guests took seats around a large table. The moderator introduced himself, made a short introductory speech, and then suggested that we should introduce ourselves, "since we are new to each other." The first physician stood and identified himself as "Carroll Leevy, New Jersey." A little sheepishly, the roll call proceeded counterclockwise around the table. "Reynolds, Los Angeles, Klatskin, New Haven, Zimmerman, Washington," etc. Each person stood and, I thought, tried not to smile. It seemed somehow to take on a more serious tone than had been intended. As the introductions approached my place between Fenton Schaffner and Hans Popper, I was struck by the ridiculousness of a bunch of people formally introducing themselves to other people whom they knew quite well. "Fenton Schaffner, New York." Suddenly, it was my turn. Almost without thinking I stood and said, "Poppa, New York" and sat down. There was a quiet murmur of laughter. Hans, who was next, stood and looked at me, a little amused and a little uncertain. As he paused with all eyes on him and his on me, I realized that he was struggling to recall my name. After a second or so, he asked quietly, "Vat *is* my name?" Even at a loss for words he knew exactly what to say.

We will all miss him in different ways.

9

Helmut Denk, Graz

MY WAY TO PATHOLOGY AND HEPATOLOGY

HANS POPPER AND VIENNA (FROM 1903 TO 1938)   The year 1938 brought a severe and irreversible loss to Austrian cultural and scientific life: Hans Popper left the country he loved and the environment that had molded him. As he told me in nightly hours when teaching me liver biopsy interpretation, life was not always easy in Vienna in the 1930s with social and political discrepancies and errors flaring up. However, it was apparently still exciting scientifically.

Hans Popper's career was exceptional from the very beginning. It did not fit into the usual frame. He preferred biochemistry despite excellence in morphology and the invitation of the famous and critical anatomist Julius Tandler to work in his department, a rare distinction for a student at that time. Later, in the Department of Pathology in Vienna, Hans Popper again went beyond the limits of the traditional autopsy-oriented discipline and employed biochemical methodology in his work, thus anticipating molecular pathology (see Fig. 9 in photo section). When he was invited to join the staff of H. Eppinger at the First Department of Internal Medicine in Vienna, he by far excelled his fellow clinicians in his struggle for scientific truth. Immediately after the war, he supported Austrian scientists and thus invaluably contributed to scientific progress in our country. The honorary doctorate of the University of Vienna on the occasion of its 600th anniversary was an attempt to acknowledge his contributions to Austrian science. For me, working for many years in the same wards and laboratories in the Departments of Internal Medicine and Pathology as Hans Popper did 30 years earlier, his name was always synonymous with innovation and scientific progress. From 1969 to 1971 I had the privilege of working with him at Mount Sinai and this determined my professional life.

HANS POPPER AND MY WAY TO PATHOLOGY   When I finished medical school, pathologic anatomy in Vienna was a highly respected discipline but, at least in my opinion, too static and conservative to be able to significantly contribute to the advancement of science. The exciting and innovative times when scientists like Karl Landsteiner and later Hans Popper worked in this department had passed. Therefore, when I decided to apply for a fellowship from the National Institutes of Health in 1969 after 2½ years of training in experimental and internal medicine, I wanted to learn the basis of liver disease in Hans Popper's department but I did not intend to become a pathologist. However, my opinion was almost immediately changed when I started work in New York. Hans Popper, his department, and, particularly, the pathology he represented were addictive. He not only kept his fellows busy almost day and night (". . . I am doing my experiments with the feet on the table; you, guys, now prove or disprove what I am saying. . . ."), but he also created an atmosphere of clinically and patient-oriented pathology combined with humanity in his research meetings, slide interpretations, autopsy rounds, and clinical–pathologic conferences that was irresistible and forced all of us to imitate. In addition, though, he was a humorous person who enjoyed the scientific and social aspects equally. So, during my fellowship in New York, I decided to devote my future professional life to pathology. After my return to Vienna, I was accepted as assistant in the Department of Pathology, which had been taken over by J.H. Holzner, a former student of Hans Popper. My Laboratory of Molecular Pathology was then dedicated to Hans Popper (Hans-Popper-Laboratory).

HANS POPPER AND MALLORY BODY RESEARCH   As a person who grew up in the Austrian environment with its positive as well as negative facets (both also pertinent to alcohol), Hans Popper always kept a sincere interest in the theory and practice of alcohol and related matters, as every Austrian and particularly Viennese does. The "Heurige" (retail of new wine) is still a characteristic feature of Viennese social life together with the *white* Lippizzaner horses, the "Sängerknaben" (boy singers), and St. Stephen's Cathedral. It could, therefore, be expected that besides cholestasis, alterations of endoplasmic reticulum, hepatitis, and liver immunology ethanol attracted considerable interest in Hans Popper's department. Studies were not restricted to rats and baboons, but from time to time a heroic autoexperiment was urgent in an effort to advance scientific progress by personal experience. In 1970, one of the first Falk Meetings was devoted to "Alcohol and

Liver" (liver during days, alcohol at nights). In this context, two facts important for my future work should be recalled. One was the notion of Fenton Schaffner that the Mallory body (MB) could serve as Rosetta stone helpful in deciphering the mystery of the pathogenesis of alcoholic liver cell damage in alcoholic hepatitis. The other, and most important, was the summary of the meeting brilliantly (as ever) delivered by Hans Popper in which be challenged the speakers of the meeting by making the injurious effects of alcohol uncertain on the basis of the scientific evidence presented. This provocation (together with some frustration) was a major stimulus for me to start work on alcoholic liver disease in the way I learned it from Hans Popper, by proceeding through several steps: (1) study of the morphology; (2) experimental reproduction of characteristic features of the disease, e.g., of MBs in suitable animals; (3) characterization of the human and experimental lesion by application of every suitable methodology, including molecular biologic techniques; and (4) interpretation of the results in a more general context.

WORK ON THE NATURE AND PATHOGENISIS OF MBs: A TRIBUTE TO HANS POPPER   In 1970, Hans Popper aroused my immediate interest in the MB when he stimulated me together with Michael Gerber and Bill Orr to study the appearance and significance of MBs in a variety of nonalcoholic liver disorders (finally published in *Gastroenterology*). Since then, we and others have made some progress concerning the nature of these peculiar inclusions, although many details still await clarification.

1. *The model.* MBs can be easily produced and studied under defined conditions in mice by prolonged administration of the antimicrotubular agent griseofulvin or of DDC. Although the ensuing liver disorder, which is associated with protoporphyria, differs in several aspects from classic alcoholic hepatitis in man, experimentally produced MBs resemble in their light—as well as electron microscopic appearance (filamentous ultrastructure)—those associated with human liver disease. This indicates that they may share a common or at least similar terminal pathogenetic pathway.

2. *The nature of MBs.* Immunohistochemical and biochemical studies revealed a close relationship between MBs and the hepatocellular keratin intermediate filament cytoskeleton. However, there are considerable structural modifications of keratins in MBs due to cross-linking, proteolysis as well as associated proteins of nonkeratin nature, including ubiquitin, as revealed by immunohistochemistry using poly- and monoclonal antibodies, gel electrophoresis, immunoblotting, column chromatography, and peptide mapping. Thus, the MB is complex and not simply the result of collapse or aggregation of intermediate filaments, and MB filaments are not what they seem to be at first glance. They are certainly intermediate in dimensions, yet not classic intermediate filaments. Activation of Ca^{2+}-dependent enzymes in

chronically injured cells could play an important role in MB pathogenesis. Partial proteolysis of hepatocytic keratins by Ca^{2+}-dependent neutral proteases followed by transglutaminase-induced cross-linking and ϵ-(γ-glutamyl) lysine-dipeptide formation may be involved. Since similar mechanisms play a role in apoptosis and amyloid formation, MB pathogenesis seems to mimick these processes to a certain degree.

3. *From liver to brain.* Filementous and tubular ultrastructure, insolubility, relationship to the intermediate filament cytoskeleton, ubiquitination, cross-linking, partial proteolytic breakdown, and association with chronic cell injuries are not unique to MBs. They are also features of a diversity of degenerative inclusion bodies, including amyloid-like structures associated with neurons in Alzheimer's disease, Pick's disease, and Parkinson's disease. Consequently, from studies of liver disease and MBs we may learn more about structure and function of the cytoskeleton in general and principles and pathways of its regulation under physiologic and pathologic conditions, not only in the liver.

OUTLOOK   Innumerable hepatologists of all fields of interest were inspired and constantly stimulated by Hans Popper. Through them future generations will carry further his scientific enthusiasm, aimed at understanding liver disease by integration of pathology, clinical experience, biochemistry, and molecular biology. His admonishment, "Let's go to work, gentlemen . . ." (as he used to say at 10 p.m. after a whole day of work in the laboratory or at the microscope), will always be an obligation to us.

10

V. J. Desmet, Leuven

I chose to illustrate my personal recollections of Hans Popper with a picture that is anything but academic (see Fig. 10 in photo section): a photograph of Hans conducting—for sheer fun—the brass orchestra during the festive evening closing the social program of one of the many symposia he conceived with Dr. Herbert Falk: "Collagen Metabolism in the Liver" held in Freiburg, Germany, in October 1973. I like this photograph because it illustrates quite well what Dr. Popper meant to me and symbolizes in a pleasant way what he meant to the field of hepatology.

I came to know Hans Popper in quite an indirect way. I graduated from medical school in Leuven in 1957, a period when growth in histopathology was dormant. My mentor in those days was Prof. Josue Vandenbroucke, chairman of the Department of Medicine at the University Hospital in Leuven and gastroenterologist with a keen interest in liver disease. It was he who finally influenced my turning to histopathology and who helped to cultivate my interest in the liver, by providing me with a newly published book, *Liver: Structure and Function*, written by two major gods of the medical Olympus from far-away America and totally unknown to me: Hans Popper and Fenton Schaffner. This was my first indirect contact with Hans Popper.

I went for training in pathology to Paris and London, carrying with me during those 2 years the "Popper book," like a bible. It must have had some influence, since, on my return to Leuven in 1959, I decided to start scientific work in no other area than experimental liver carcinogenesis.

The growing interest in structure and function of the normal and diseased liver made me search for every paper written in those years by Popper and associates. I was amazed and fascinated by their various attempts at correlating structure and function. Their approach contrasted considerably with much of the descriptive pathology of that and earlier times.

The conviction grew that Popper's approach to liver histopathology was the right and only way to practice histopathology: by continuously searching for structural–functional relationships in health and disease. This concept was enforced by the marvelous results appearing at that time in the burgeoning fields of histochemistry, cell fractionation, and electron microscopy. So strong was the obsession by my "prototype" that Prof. Vandenbroucke, by then dean of our medical school, was easily convinced to nominate that fabulous American pathologist for an honorary degree at the Catholic University of Leuven. Maybe the dean already had his own opinion, but I prefer to believe I had some influence.

My first encounter with Hans Popper was in 1965 when he came to Leuven to receive his "doctor honoris causa" charter: I was his driver, in charge of taking him from Brussels to the ceremony at the university promotion hall in Leuven. The next day, he paid a visit to my laboratory and had some time to talk. This brief encounter deepened my previous desire to join his famous group, hoping to pursue some worthwhile work with him.

However, local circumstances kept me here. I had become submerged in routine diagnostic work as recently appointed head of the local department of pathology and was drowning in endless teaching obligations for far too many students. That was it then: I had a job and had to pay for it. I would not work with Popper, I would not be his student, and I would not have my name appearing on his papers.

In 1968, results of some histochemical endeavors brought me to the Congress of Histochemistry and Cytochemistry in New York. On this occasion, Dr. and Mrs. Popper—through Dr. Tibor Barka, who had located me during a session in the meeting room—invited me for dinner at their home. I will always remember that special evening, which allowed me to discover a friendly, warm, and entertaining man behind the Popper of my books and papers.

In the meantime, a group of European clinicians and pathologists with interest in liver disease had clung together since their first encounter during the second EASL meeting in Göteborg in 1967 and had worked on a new classification of chronic hepatitis, which was formulated in Zürich in 1968. This achievement procured the nickname "gnomes of Zürich" from Dame Sheila Sherlock, who named the group this way during her speech at the congress banquet of the IASL meeting in Karlovy Vary in 1968. The nickname would become, in later years, a label of prestige.

From their very start, the "gnomes" had the intention to have Hans Popper as a member of the group: he was the foremost influential liver pathologist, and, after all, a European, like the rest of us. Formally invited after our Zürich meeting in 1968, Hans Popper sent his representative to the 1969 meeting in Leuven, but when it dawned on him that this was not what was expected from a "gnome," he decided to attend the next meeting in person.

I remember the slight nervousness among a few of us, when our host Hemming Poulsen guided the group to the meeting room in Kommune Hospitalet in Copenhagen the afternoon of Tuesday, July 7th, 1970. Without Popper, we already had gone through three working rounds the previous years, had come to know each other fairly well, and were already used to frank and free discussion. How would it be when the shadow of this superman loomed over us? Could one still be fair and show one's ignorance in front of him, who knew it all? Would it be wise to speak at all, or—even worse—to disagree? Any apprehensions we had soon dissipated; it did not take long before we felt at home with him, and he apparently with us.

For 17 more years, Hans Popper was the heart, the motor, and the spirit of these meetings. Browsing through my notes from these fantastic 3-day-long discussions causes nostalgia to set in and revives many vivid images. I hear him cite again those long-forgotten papers and mention the most recent ones (to be published in a future issue of a journal he reviewed) (see Fig. 11 in photo section) . . . I see him at the blackboard, drawing portal tracts and "bridges," lymphocytes, and fibers, right across the list of items just tabulated for discussion. I see him striding up and down, gesturing broadly, supporting firm argumentation . . . or leaning back with half-closed eyes when citing data from experiments "way back in the fifties" . . . or jumping up to talk for half an hour to a group of baffled "gnomes," explaining with excitement the hottest news in the exploding field of collagen research or on eicosanoids in inflammation. In later years, I see him dozing off awhile when the discussion drifts toward the other side, only to make a crucial remark or to produce the sought-after answer when he apparently wakes up again.

Every "gnome," for sure, agrees that he learned enormously from him, but Hans went on pretending that he was learning from us all and that this meeting was the best each year (he never skipped a single one).

He was the true conductor of that chamber orchestra of "gnomes"; he knew the scores by heart, astonishing us all with his unfailing memory; he knew the art of interpreting a difficult passage and had the gift to stimulate crescendos by his visions and dreams; he had authority, charisma, fantasy; he would criticize, encourage, and correct, aiming at perfection . . . all gifts that made him a remarkable conductor. The papers we wrote together were a tremendous exercise with Popper as composer. He was guiding, correcting, and inspiring all the time.

Hans Popper also was composer and conductor for far larger groups than the "gnomes." He was the very best "maestro" at innumerable huge meetings (suffice it to refer to the Basel Liver Weeks (Fig. 12), the Chicago meetings, and World Congresses) and composer of those special programs that he termed "experiments in communication" intended to expose hepatologists to basic science and vice versa.

He was incredibly creative and profuse in producing scientific compositions. There is no need to list his hundreds of published papers, the chapters and books, the research units, the new medical school, the nationwide and worldwide associations that resulted from his mind and from his work. All these have amply been reviewed in festschrifts or reiterated at the celebrations marking his 70th, 75th, and 80th birthdays. (These were, in fact, my sources to learn of Popper's past.)

Some performances have left exceptionally deep impressions. One still marvels at his sparkling fantasy, expressed in a remarkably refreshing way with nostalgic undertones, in his famous talk, "Vienna and the Liver," on the occasion of the celebration of his 80th birthday in the Vienna of his youth. Who among the hundreds who were there will easily forget his mastery of modern science, demonstrated by his impressive closing lecture in Basel in 1982 ending the meeting, "Structural Carbohydrates in the Liver," with the crowded audience in an immense lecture hall rising to their feet for a thunderous standing ovation?

These, then, are some of the reasons why I like that photograph of Hans from 1973. It portrays a conductor! It also shows him as the smiling, joyful man he was.

Over the years, from the time he joined the "gnomes" in 1970, I came to know him better after countless chats and talks at coffee breaks and over drinks and dinner: he became a good, close friend.

Not only did he strike me with his restless drive for knowledge, he also was a most attractive model of a human being, a highly cultured man who took pleasure in living. He also had a taste for the best in life, including fine food and superior wine. He was a pleasant, joyful master.

I am not sure whether he had special musical gifts or talents (I will have to read another biographical sketch). But I am sure of this: that he was the universally acclaimed "maestro" of the great unfinished symphony entitled "international hepatology." Notwithstanding some despair in early years, it was my privilege to be his student in some way, to work with him, and to have my name on some of his important writings.

11

Herbert Falk, Freiburg

I met Hans and Lina Popper in 1965 in Basel. Kurt Beck and I had the pleasure of picking them up at the Hotel Trois Rois and to drive them to Freiburg. There they were visiting Prof. Ludwig Heilmeyer whom they had seen a few days before in Vienna, where both men had received honorary degrees on the occasion of the 600th anniversary of the founding of the university. Both men also held honorary degrees from the Catholic University of Leuven. The Heilmeyers, Poppers, Becks, and I had lunch at the restaurant Zur Traube in the old part of Freiburg, and then Hans gave a lecture at the medical school of the university for the house staff and students. This accidental meeting led to a 23-year-long relationship of active and far-reaching cooperation nobody could have foreseen. We met again 1 year later at the World Congress of Gastroenterology in Tokyo and at the succeeding meeting of the IASL in Kyoto and again found many mutual interests that subsequently led to close collaboration and friendship.

FALK SYMPOSIA   Our initial cooperation resulted in the first Falk Symposium in October 1967. Ludwig Heilmeyer (see Fig. 13 in photo section) was president, although he had left Freiburg and had moved to Ulm as the founding dean of the newly created medical school. The meeting was organized by Kurt Beck (unfortunately now also deceased), well counseled and advised by Hans. At that time, my firm was rather small, and we expected about 200–300 attendees. However, 800 physicians came from 17 countries, and I will never forget that the 3-day meeting cost me half of my 1967 turnover. From 1970 to 1987 there were 24 Falk Symposia dominated by Hans and greatly influenced by his knowledge, intelligence, and experience. Organization and execution of these meetings followed a certain pattern: Hans had good ideas for topics and subjects and always knew the right and best people whom we could approach as planners and organizers. It took many transatlantic phone calls to decide the referees until everything was to his liking. When all was said and done, the programs were outstanding, and many physicians and scientists from all over the globe honored the meetings with their presence. Thus, the Falk Symposia guided by Hans (24 plus one posthumously) were attended by 19,000 participants from about 70 countries. Hans was either president, scientific organizer, or moderator; sometimes he functioned as all three. When he was in charge, there was always an interesting, lively, and stimulating discussion, which often ended in ovations for him that lasted minutes. Without question, the high point was Falk Symposium No. 39 in October 1983 in Vienna, his birthplace, on the occasion of his 80th birthday; 650 attended from 34 countries. He opened the meeting himself with his original and clever paper, "Vienna and the Liver." The audience was deeply moved, and one of his co-workers, Dr. Swan Thung, had to interrupt her own subsequent talk because she was so moved. Hans received a prestigious medal from the Minister of Culture: a high decoration for Science and Art, First Class of the Republic of Austria (Ehrenzeichen für Wissenschaft und Kunst).

The first Basel Liver Week without Hans took place in 1989 (Nos. 54 and 55). However, 2 years before, he had put down his ideas as to the topic and the composition of the organizing committee. It was a big success, but the 1,400 participants missed him. On this occasion, the first Hans Popper Award was given to Prof. Thomas of London, and it was the fourth time that the Hans Popper Promotion Prize (Förderpreis) was given to a young German-speaking scientist.

HEPATOLOGY RAPID LITERATURE REVIEW Another venture of our collaboration was the Hepatology Rapid Literature Review, first published in 1971, appearing monthly since then. This publication collects and prints abstracts from 600 medical journals from all over the world; on the average, there are 8,000 abstracts annually. The international hepatology community welcomes and happily subscribes to it. The initial difficulties, mainly of a legal nature, were soon overcome and with a minimum of red tape, thanks to Hans' many friends in the right places. Subsequently, at the end of each year, Hans wrote an "Abstract of Abstracts," in which he summarized the most important and promising scientific information of the year on about 40 typewritten pages after thoroughly weighing and critically rating all 8,000 publications. This "Abstract of Abstracts" was partly translated into German and Japanese and was an important tool and resource material. Here, too, he leaves a vacuum.

MEDICAL POSTGRADUATE MEETINGS AND CONGRESSES IN EUROPE Between 1970 and 1987, Hans spoke at innumerable medical postgraduate courses, meetings, symposia, and congresses in all of Europe. I often accompanied and chauffeured him around to the various places. He was always a lively companion, and we often had animated, sometimes heated, discussions. Speed and heavy traffic on the autobahn presented hazards, and it was often strenuous for me. The daily schedule of those trips was mostly the same: leave the hotel early in the morning and drive several hundred kilometers to arrive punctually at the next location. In university towns, Hans always wanted to visit the medical schools to discuss science and exchange information with the young house staff in a small circle. He always said that he learned at least as much from them as they learned from him. The postgraduate events usually took place in the late afternoon or early evening, and his talks were invariably well received, with great enthusiasm and much applause. As a rule, the size of the audience was between 100 and 500. Ordinarily, there was a "gemütlich" get-together afterwards, often lasting until late because many wanted to talk to Hans and ask him questions; he always responded with great patience and forbearance. This, however, did not keep him from getting up the next morning 1 or 2 hours earlier than his much younger companions in order to do his Canadian Air Force exercises. These trips took us up and down through West Germany, through Switzerland, Italy, Austria, Yugoslavia, France, Belgium, Holland, Great Britain, Hungary, and Czechoslovakia as well as East Germany. Two events will stay with me for a long time.

In October 1980, a Collagen Metabolism congress took place at the University of Münster. The meeting started Thursday morning, but Hans' schedule showed a lecture in Heidelberg the night before. Therefore, the organizers of the Münster meeting arranged that Hans would arrive there about noon. All was well planned, but we did not count on Hans. He insisted to be driven to Münster after his talk in Heidelberg in order to arrive punctually at the beginning of the meeting. It was well after midnight when my co-worker, Klaus Gärtner, drove the 77-year-old man 500 kilometers, arriving in Münster early in the morning. At 9 a.m., Hans sat happily in his seat in the first row.

Another story stays in my mind: it happened in May 1984 on a visit to East Berlin. Hans had to lecture 250 attendees in the Hotel Intercontinental in West Berlin. The next morning he, his wife and mine, my daughter Carola, and I took the S Bahn from the Zoo Station in West Berlin across the sector border to the Friedrichstrasse Station in East Berlin. At that point, the border control was very strict. We stood in a very dark and narrow corridor, one behind the other. Through a tiny slit the harsh voice of an invisible bureaucrat demanded our passports. We stood in uncomfortable silence. Hans who had fled Hitler's Austria in 1938 knew the importance of a valid passport, the lack of which sometimes was a matter of life and death. Thus, even the relatively short time this document was in the hands of the East German VOPO made him nervous and edgy. We all understood and sympathized. Our East German colleagues awaited us and took us to the Charité, the hospital of the Humboldt University. There Hans was greeted with great enthusiasm, which he obviously cherished after the unpleasant excitement at the border. A few East Berlin physicians took us on a rather long trip around West Berlin in order to get to Potsdam, which lay only a few kilometers away as the crow flies. There as almost everywhere in Europe, Hans remembered his first visit to Potsdam with his parents and grandparents. That evening all of us were more than happy to find ourselves back in West Germany.

He absolutely broke the record of his lecture activities in October 1985. Between October 5th and 17th, Hans gave 10 talks in 10 different places in West Germany, Switzerland, and Austria; all in all he talked to 2,500 people. That was when I drove him 3,300 kilometers. The conclusion of this trip was a congress in Brescia, North Italy. The following year, at Lina's suggestion, travel was somewhat curtailed. In 1987, he gave several talks in Germany and also received his last honorary degree from the University of Göttingen. Hannover, Münster, and Freiburg had honored him some years before as did 10 other universities in Europe. Unfortunately, the offer of an honorary degree from the Humboldt University in East Berlin came at a time when Hans was already quite sick. His last European trip was in the fall of 1987, and I will talk about it later.

HANS AND "VACATIONS" The frequency and length of vacations that he permitted himself in the last 20 years can be compared to the time off Japanese high executives take, i.e., he hardly ever took any, and if so they lasted 1 or 2 days, much to Lina's regret. Before coming to Europe in 1983, he informed me that he absolutely wanted to take 2 days off, in a very nice place in Switzerland, at least five stars. He wanted to pay for it, but he wanted me to choose it. I was worried when I picked up Hans and Lina in Zurich with a small list of potential places. First, I took them to Brunnen on the Vierwaldstätter See, where we lunched at the Hotel Waldstätter Hof. However, despite five stars the place did not meet expectations, and so we went around the lake along the Burgenstock, but that five-star hotel was also out of the question because there was no indoor pool. We crossed the Bruning Pass and arrived at Interlaken. The hotel where he would have liked to stay, the Victoria Jungfrau, where he had stayed as a child with his parents, was unfortunately full with a cardiology meeting. Swissair had helped me to reserve a lovely suite in the neighboring four-star Hotel Metropole. But, as Hans saw this very modern, square cement block, he put thumbs down and said he wanted to see something else. Thanks to the kind help of Fred Halter and his wife, we finally drove to the last of the five-star places on my list, the Hotel Beatus in Merligen on Lake Thun. Worriedly, I got out of the car wondering whether this place would fulfill Hans' idea of Nirvana or Shangri-la for 2 days. Eureka! He thought it was ideal, and I jumped for joy. While the Poppers checked in, I called the Hotel Metropole in Interlaken to cancel the reservation. The receptionist was quite upset and asked what to do with the beautiful flowers that were already waiting. I generously offered them to her and after dinner drove happily home to Freiburg.

ASIA TRIP WITH HANS IN 1986   In January of 1986, I planned a lengthy trip to Asia with Hans, Lina, and my friend, Peter Maier of Esslingen. We met in Singapore for the annual Asian Pacific ASL. As usual, Hans dominated the meeting, which was held at the very pleasant Shangri-la Hotel, where all of us stayed. On January 12th we drove through the jungle to Kuala Lumpur, the capital of Malaysia, and then returned to Singapore by plane. The next morning we went to Jakarta, the capital of Indonesia. Hans gave a talk at the university in terrible heat, and he was continuously interrupted by ice pieces falling from the air conditioner, the thermostat of which was as high as it would go. Then we went to Shanghai. Prof. Tang was the president of the International Congress on Liver Cancer and Hepatitis, held January 15–17. In contrast to hot Indonesia, Shanghai was very cold. Neither the old Shanghai Hotel nor the congress building were heated, although the temperature was just above zero. But Chinese rules say buildings can only be heated when the outside temperature is below zero. At the opening of the meeting, the Europeans and the Americans sat shivering in their seats. The mayor of the town in his down coat counseled wisely "to generate heat through our enthusiasm for the science of hepatology and thus warm the hall."

Through the literature Hans had learned that the highest incidence of hepatitis B and liver cancer occurred in the Southern provinces of China, especially in Nanning. Of course, we had to visit there despite the winter weather and the enormous distance. So our small group flew to Guilin with our excellent translator, Prof. Wang. The Hotel Lijang was only partly occupied because of reconstruction. A delegation of pathologists from the provincial capital had taken an overnight trip by train and were already waiting for us. They had arrived 2 days ahead of time to be sure to meet the famous professor and discuss science with him. Since the days were devoted to sightseeing, especially a boat ride on the beautiful Lijang River, the research discussions took place at night. There was a shortage of rooms, so they talked in the room of my friend, Peter Maier. All worked very hard without letup to communicate and to exchange information about the importance of hepatitis and liver cell cancer. The talks lasted until long after midnight. However, I am not sure whether the Chinese doctors understood all that those two tried so hard to explain, whether their English was really adequate. After 2 days, we returned to Shanghai in an old Russian plane and after a short stay there we flew on to Tokyo and to the good old, well-heated Okura Hotel. It felt like we had landed on another planet. Under Hans' guidance, a symposium, "New Trends in Hepatology," took place in Tokyo (January 24th and 25th). Our little group had traveled to five countries in 18 days, from tropical heat in Indonesia to the cold in unheated Shanghai.

HANS' LAST EUROPEAN TRIP   His last trip was in October 1987 involving talks and meetings in Italy and Germany. Hans and Lina arrived in Kloten on October 11th; I picked them up, and, as so many times before, we drove south through the Gotthard Tunnel. In Lugano, we stayed in a lovely and beautifully situated hotel, the Principe Leopoldo. The next morning, Hans visited the University of Milan; he spoke there in the evening at a medical meeting and the next afternoon he spoke in Bologna. On the afternoon of October 13th, we drove along the Adriatic Sea to Ancona, where the annual Italian ASL met. For the day before, they had organized an extraordinary presentation in a little town in the Abbruzzi. A medical school was founded in Chieti only in the 1980s. The University of Bologna acted as the god-father to this new school. The chairmen of the departments lived and worked mainly in Bologna and spent only 1 or 2 days a week in Chieti. The faculty was interested in giving special importance and validity to this still-unknown and unproven institution by the visit of a man of Hans' reputation. When we first heard of this plan we asked everybody, "Where is Chieti?" After a lot of telephoning back and forth, we finally found this little place on the map, and Hans immediately agreed to go. Actually, this was very characteristic of him. If asked to speak, he hardly ever said no, no matter how large or small, near or far the place might be. A co-worker of mine, Dr. Pappini, drove us through the Marches. We stopped at the Shrine of Loretto, but despite the beauty of the old buildings Hans was very upset at the sight of the many sick people who sought miracle cures. Therefore, we left soon and drove south along the Adriatic Sea to Pescara and then inland into the mountains to Chieti. The school was still under construction, and it was difficult to get around. However, it was a red-letter day for the Chieti faculty and students, and, despite the dust, Hans talked to a large and appreciative group. We returned to Ancona the same night, and Hans participated in the meeting. On October 18th, we returned to Germany, specifically to Munich. I had planned a direct and fast route through Bologna, Verona, and Bozen, but Hans had found out that Lina had never been in the Dolomites. This was a valid reason to make a detour via Padua and Treviso and then upstream the Piave River towards Cortina. There was hardly any traffic because it was between seasons. We reached Cortina in the early afternoon, driving the many hundreds of curves of the Dolomite Road over the many passes. We stopped for lunch and went via the Grödner Valley to the Brenner autobahn. Dusk fell, it started to rain, and finally we arrived tired but gratified in Munich. A postgraduate course was planned for the next day in which Drs. Deinhardt and Paumgartner participated, and it was, as usual, well attended. There followed a medical program in Cologne, and in Frankfurt 350 fascinated physicians listened to him. Hans and Lina then flew to Amsterdam. On October 23, Hans gave his last European lecture in Rotterdam in Prof. Schalm's department. My wife used to call these trips "barnstorming tours." Hans loved to have contact with as many people as possible, to stimulate and be stimulated; then he was in his glory. For me these travels to meetings and congresses were a continuous source of inspiration, and I will never forget them.

12

Stephen A. Geller, Los Angeles

H ans Popper was just a name I knew as the "pathologist-in-chief" of The Mount Sinai Hospital when I came to see him in the spring of 1964 to be interviewed for a first-year residency position in pathology. Although I had decided to study pathology while still a medical student, I was remarkably lacking in knowledge about the nuances of residency programs. On the advice of some of the pathologists and other physicians at Lenox Hill Hospital, where I was a rotating intern, I applied to Albert Einstein, Kings County, Lenox Hill, and Mount Sinai.

My interview with Dr. Popper was preceded by a tour of the department with one of the younger staff pathologists, who assured me that there were "50 or 60" applicants for the first-year positions. The interview with Dr. Popper was relatively brief. I was overwhelmed by the grandeur of his office with its palpable air of knowledge and energy, the walls of books, the honorary degrees, the many photographs, but especially by the graciousness of the man who I had a little trouble understanding. Two specifics about that first meeting are etched forever indelibly in my memory, however. First, he assured me that I could come to Mount Sinai as a resident if I decided to do so. Few events have been so flattering to me as that invitation, inflating my ego far beyond what it deserved. Second, he asked me if I would mind going from his office, on the fourth floor of the Atran Building, to the "E" level to meet with Dr. Otani. Anticipating my confusion, he told me that Dr. Otani was a great pathologist who was very senior, and, although Dr. Otani did not really take part in selecting new residents, he, Hans Popper, would be most grateful if I would take a few minutes to meet with Dr. Otani. I never fail to smile when I think of that generosity and warmth of spirit that led

Hans Popper, internationally recognized physician and scientist, to ask if he could impose on me, still drenching wet behind the ears, to meet Sadao Otani. I'm not sure how much I understood at that moment how these two human beings, each extraordinary in his own way, would influence my whole life.

As I think of Hans Popper, as I do almost every day because his picture is in my office right above my desk, there is a flood of memories, a confusing wealth of images, thoughts, and feelings, still warm, still inspiring, still guiding, still overwhelming, and still a little bit intimidating.

Somehow it has only been since he died that I have been able to devote myself largely to hepatic pathology. I can only label myself "liver pathologist" today without too much hesitancy. When Hans Popper was alive I never had the *chutzpah* to do that.

After the first few months of my pathology residency, I was quite unhappy and considered quitting. I have since learned that this is not an uncommon reaction among neophytes as they watch staff members seemingly able to see the history of the world in each histologic section, and more senior residents able to see at least the major events. I was particularly discouraged by watching Dr. Popper in action. Was this what a pathologist is supposed to do? Study a single organ from a complicated autopsy and tell the patient's age, sex, metabolic state, and diagnoses; see things in liver biopsy slides that no one else quite discerned, and do it in the often flickering glare of a carbon-arc projector while drinking coffee with one hand, rummaging through the pockets of the laboratory coat looking for a match with the other hand, relighting the uncooperative and ever-present (in those days) pipe with another hand, and pointing to the key histologic feature with yet another hand; publish landmark and insightful papers seemingly every day; lecture at medical schools and scientific assemblies around the world; evaluate innumerable consultation slides, also from around the world; lead a busy and productive clinical department; manage a busy and even more productive research team; create a medical school; be an acknowledged and actively practicing expert pathologist, anatomist, physiologist, biochemist, geneticist, gastroenterologist, social and medical historian, health-care planner; found a subspecialty; work from early morning to late at night every day except Saturday, when you could go home for dinner, and Sunday, when you could go home at noon; and, fortunately for so many of us, devote untold hours to neophyte pathologists; and even more. It was only when I realized that no other pathologist, no other person, in the world could do all these things that I was able to overcome my concerns and continue with my career.

After a trip, usually covering at least three major world cities in as many days with at least two lectures per city, Dr. Popper would sweep into the old residents' room on his first day back to find out what was new. Some fresh, uninitiated resident might ask, "Were you on vacation, Dr. Popper?" His reply was distinctive both for the accent and the consistent response: "Ya, I was playing golf!" Once, when I was a senior resident, I happened to look out the window of the Atran Surgical Pathology Laboratory and saw Dr. Popper on Madison Avenue, with a small suitcase, trying to flag down a cab. It was approximately 9:30 in the morning and I had finished with my cases. I ran down and asked him if I could drive him somewhere. He had to get to LaGuardia Airport for a trip to Chicago. He accepted my offer, letting me know he had a 10 o'clock flight, and I ran down 98th Street to retrieve my Volkswagen "beetle." To say that I drove like a madman would be a generous understatement. We pulled up to the terminal at approximately 9:55. I apologized profusely for getting him there so close to departure time and expressed my hope that he would not miss his plane. "I am so grateful to you, Dr. Geller," he said, "you have been most kind, and I have never been here so early before!"

After my residency, I fulfilled my Berry Plan military obligation at the Naval Hospital, in Beaufort, South Carolina. My wife and I left New York in 1969 vowing never to return, to head out for new frontiers. Periodically I would write a short social letter to Dr. Popper, and he would always graciously reply. He took time to encourage me to obtain a faculty position at the medical school in Charleston and wrote a letter, and made a phone call, on my behalf. This was a double-edged sword, of course. Although I was made most welcome in Gordon Hennigar's excellent department, I was also expected to demonstrate, on a regular basis, that I was a Popper-taught hepatopathologist.

After the first year in Beaufort, I started to apply for staff positions in a number of cities: Houston, Boston, Atlanta. I was especially interested in a small Boston hospital, affiliated with Harvard. I submitted a letter and spoke to the incumbent pathologist, who was planning to retire. He invited me to send some dates for an interview. A few weeks later he called me, quite irate, to ask why I was wasting his valuable time, since Dr. Popper had just informed him that I was coming back to Mount Sinai. Until that moment, I had not considered rejoining the department, but immediately came to the realization that there was nothing else I wanted to do but come back to New York and to the department that was home for me, with those marvelous teachers who made pathology a rich and vibrant and exciting way of life, rather than a job: Sadao Otani, Lotte Strauss, Jack Churg, Fenton Schaffner, Fred Zak, Mamoru Kaneko, Cyril Toker, Fiorenzo Paronetto, David Koffler, Emanuel Rubin, and, leading this disparate group of talented and dynamic pathologists, Hans Popper.

The Saturday morning conferences are forever etched in my memory. A packed room, with pathologists coming from a number of hospitals around the city to the Saturday autopsy presentation conference, presented by first-year residents but presided over by Popper and Otani, with the other staff members actively contributing, sometimes to the distress of the presenter. With almost 600 autopsies that first year of my residency, we were busy and learning more than we could appreciate at the time. I can still see the room in total darkness (no rheostats for the lights, then), one of us at the screen, another struggling to keep the carbons of the projector close enough together to emit light but not close enough to fuse, while Dr. Popper pointed to some key area with the stem of his pipe. A few years later he would take delight in whipping out his telescoping pointer for that purpose.

We each presented a case almost every Saturday. It was the task of the one who was least occupied with presentations to prepare Dr. Popper's coffee. At the back of the room, we had a Bunsen burner under a tripod support on which sat a tea kettle. A key trick was to turn off the burner as soon as the water boiled, but before it whistled. A jar of instant coffee was the necessary reagent. Once, in the first weeks of my first year, when I was a very young, very meek, very insecure resident, it was my turn to make Dr. Popper's coffee. I managed very well getting the granules of coffee into the cup, turning off the fire at the right moment, and pouring the boiling water into the cup. Unfortunately, I temporarily lost "sight" of the cup in the dark room while I put the very hot pot back on the support. When I reached for the cup I spilled it on my then ample midsection. I can still feel the heat penetrating my lab coat and my clothes and can almost hear my own muffled "ohhhhhhh" as I tried not to make a sound, since Dr. Popper was now up at the screen pacing back and forth in and out of the light as he discussed systemic lupus while I developed a non-lupoid "rash."

Dr. Popper and the Kodak carousel slide projector did not get along in the mid-1960s. He had been presenting a lecture, and one of his slides became jammed in the projector interrupting both his concentration and the delivery of his talk. Consequently, he insisted on the Leitz projector, which only accepted two slides, the one in front of the light beam and the one that would be next. The side-to-side delivery tray could not be jammed, but required a certain degree of effort on the part of the projectionist. At Dr. Popper's CPCs it was generally the task of one of the senior residents to project the slides. This was no small responsibility, since Dr. Popper tended to show many photomicrographs to illustrate a case. Every once in a while the lowly projectionist would let his concentration lag and Dr. Popper would have to say "next" a second, or even a third time. Although he never criticized any of us, there was certainly a great deal of self-castigation when the projection job was less than perfect.

The Mount Sinai Hospital CPCs were exciting and memorable. The cases were fantastic and the clinical discussions were often extraordinary. Of course, there were occasional disasters. One of the most memorable was the first Solomon Berson CPC. It was the tradition that the first CPC of the year would be presented by the chairman of pathology and the chairman of medicine. CPCs were great events and it was considered an honor to participate. For the younger clinicians and pathologists it was also a way to earn "points" on the institution reputation scale. In any event, Solomon Berson was the new chairman of medicine, having succeeded Alexander Gutman. For his first CPC he gave an elegant, thoughtful, complete, even brilliant discussion of hemobilia. Unfortunately, the clinical history he had been given contained a few "curveballs" that were not exactly accurate. For those of us who knew the case Dr. Popper had selected, it seemed as if Dr. Berson was discussing his own personal patient, and not the case for which Dr. Popper had a full tray of kodachromes. It was clear to those of us who knew him that Dr. Popper was aware that a disaster was unfolding and he began his presentation with a few remarks to try and explain how Berson might have missed the mark. He then went on to give his own elegant, thoughtful, complete, even brilliant discussion of alcoholic hepatitis.

For a period the word was that Berson thought he had been deliberately "set up." Dr. Popper was certainly embarrassed. Berson himself reviewed the chart and prepared his own version of the history, documenting those key omissions that had led him astray, and had his review distributed to the entire hospital medical staff, including interns, residents, and fellows. This, I think, prolonged Dr. Popper's embarrassment. He may also have thought that Dr. Berson's response was a little excessive. I think they became close friends and colleagues after that and worked well together up until the time of Berson's decidedly untimely death.

We were all encouraged to perform some research during those years. During my first and second years, Larry Alpert studied the effects on the rabbit liver of forced-feeding of cholesterol, and I helped him with the project. Larry prepared an abstract for the Federation meeting and we were both encouraged to go to Atlantic City for the meeting. I shall never forget Dr. Popper inviting me to the evening dinner with all the people interested in hepatology. As I came into the room he greeted me at the door and made sure to introduce me, a second-year resident, to the various professors and department chairmen in attendance.

I eventually selected cardiac pathology as an area of interest and began a fairly ambitious study of the ultrastructural features of the myocardium of patients being operated on for chronic rheumatic heart disease. The electron microscope was not available for residents during the day, certainly not if they were studying heart instead of liver, and I usually was able to get an 8 p.m. or 9 p.m. slot on the signup sheet. The electron microscope was on the fourth floor of the Atran Building at that time, not too far from Dr. Popper's office. I usually finished in about an hour, or sooner if the filament blew as it often did (I never did learn how to change the filament in that old Hitachi scope). Dr. Popper usually finished his day, in those years, at about 10, and we would meet by the elevators every now and then. I was exhausted by that time, but I don't remember ever seeing him looking fatigued until many years later when he was in his late 70s. And I only had the stamina to use the scope once, or at the most twice, a week. He, of course, was there every night. Occasionally, I would see him earlier in the evening, running up to his office from the cafeteria with the inevitable tuna sandwich in hand.

My understanding of the true meaning of graciousness, warmth, charm, and culture came, at least in large part, from the wonderful dinners at the home of Hans and Lina Popper. He never failed to radiate joy and pride as he showed his father's picture to his guests, or some memento of his life in Vienna, or a wonderful old medical book he had on his shelf. In later years, my wife and I would occasionally go out to dinner with them and he and I would walk home, a few steps behind the ladies, especially in the last few years, and we would talk. Mostly he would talk and I would listen, since I never ceased to be overwhelmed by his intelligence, kindness, wonderful wit, and thoughtfulness.

Dr. Popper came to Los Angeles during my first year here to present the annual guest lecture at the Los Angeles Society of Pathologists meeting. I also asked him to speak before our hospital medical staff. As usual, his trip was brief. About a week before he was due to come, we spoke on the phone and I apologized for squeezing in a second lecture during a short visit. What did I mean a second lecture? Is that all? He insisted that we also visit the USC Liver Unit at Rancho Los Amigos Hospital after his Cedars-Sinai lecture. I hastily arranged for that; they, of course, were delighted that he was taking the time to visit them. His lecture at Cedars-Sinai, on chronic hepatitis, was chock full of information but was somehow not quite up to his usual standard and I told myself that the years, and illness, had finally caught up with Hans Popper. He was as lively, bright, and exciting to be with as ever as we drove away from the hospital and headed for Downey, where the hospital was and where I had never been. I was so delighted to be with him and to have the opportunity to talk that I headed the wrong direction on the freeway and we landed along Santa Monica Beach.

We eventually made it to Rancho Los Amigos for some excellent discussions of a topic that was relatively new at the time, delta hepatitis, and one that he, as usual, already knew everything about and had studied extensively. His enthusiasm and energy was as it had always been and we, and they at Rancho, had a marvelous visit. That evening he spoke at the Los Angeles Society of Pathologists meeting about carcinogenesis and hepatocellular carcinoma and, again, he was dynamic and provocative, and the assembled pathologists literally bubbled with excitement at the end of his presentation. I couldn't understand why his talk at Cedars-Sinai had been so muted, but would not dare to ask him. He surely must have read my mind because he told me, when I spoke to him some weeks later, that he had experienced an attack of angina pectoris while at the podium and had trouble getting his nitroglycerin tablets. He hoped that his lecture had not been too disappointing.

On one of our last walks, during a visit I made to New York, he shared his sadness with me over the unhappy publicity that followed the proposed creation of the prize in the name of his former teacher, Eppinger. He told me of his last years in Vienna and how Eppinger had been instrumental in helping him escape the onrush of Hitler. Although he understood how Eppinger's wartime activities would require such a strong and condemning response, he could not reject someone who had been such an important influence on his life and who had helped guide him toward his career as the premier hepatologist of the world. He was deeply hurt by the criticism directed specifically against his support for the establishment of the Eppinger prize.

The research project in which I am still engaged, studying the liver pathology in a transgenic mouse model for alpha-1-antitrypsin disease, began at about the time Dr. Popper was dying. I wrote to him at about that time and asked a number of questions about the research I was beginning, knowing that his insights could lead to a thousand and one exciting avenues of investigation. Lina told me he was too sick at that time and never read the letter. I shall always be saddened that I never had the opportunity to "repay" him for all his gifts to me by presenting him with an exciting and challenging problem with which he would help me. He would have loved to provide that guidance.

Now, more than 3 years after his death, it sometimes seems as if I have not seen him for decades. Hardly a day goes by that I do not struggle with some problem in liver pathology, try to understand some sophisticated research article, or attempt to teach some young pathologist a nuance of liver pathology, all the while knowing that Dr. Popper could instantly solve the problem, decipher the article, or explain the principle better than anyone and carry out these activities with grace, wit, and authority.

13

Michael A. Gerber, New Orleans

Swan N. Thung, New York

Dr. Popper's accomplishments as teacher and educator have not always been fully recognized. He was instrumental in conceptualizing and developing The Mount Sinai School of Medicine in New York; he authored many papers on medical education and medical schools in the United States (1–12); and he taught or trained legions of medical students, residents, fellows, and pathologists, many of whom went on to successful careers and influential positions at home and abroad, including a dozen chairmen of University Departments of Pathology. In this contribution, we wish to reminisce about the day-to-day activities of Dr. Popper in teaching and in education from the perspective of his residents and fellows. The sketch on the next page shows Dr. Popper among his residents as seen through the eyes of one of them.

As chairman of the Department of Pathology, and subsequently as dean of The Mount Sinai School of Medicine, Dr. Popper was an extremely busy man. Nevertheless, he spent a significant amount of time with his residents and fellows. This was accomplished by working long hours in the hospital, usually from 8 a.m. until 10 p.m., with the exception of Saturdays and Sundays, which were ("only") 8-hour work days. More importantly, however, he used his time very effectively and exploited many of his activities for teaching purposes. His slide reviews became most instructive teaching sessions, whether conducted at his microscope or on the projection screen in

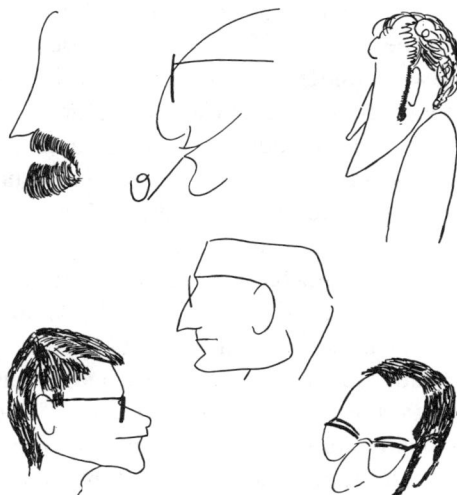

Dr. Popper (center, upper row) among his residents. (Contributed by Dr. A. Toth, New York.)

the conference room. We were prepared for a wonderful learning experience when we sat down with him and Fenton (Schaffner) at 8 p.m. or 9 p.m. to review the liver biopsy slides of the day. Without knowledge of the clinical history or laboratory data in order not to be biased, Dr. Popper would review the slides and describe the histologic findings and his thoughts in the analysis of his observations, often leading to a brilliant diagnosis, sometimes wrong, but more frequently correct when synthesized with the clinical and laboratory data. Often he would stop and say with a twinkle in his eyes, "Let me teach you something." Then he would show us a histologic finding, usually not a curious histologic alteration but a morphologic change related to the underlying pathologic condition or pathogenic mechanism.

Another treat was Dr. Popper's gross review session of the autopsies of the week. All pathology faculty members would assemble in the morgue. Dr. Popper would review the autopsy organs, again without knowledge of the clinical data. He was a master in assembling the pathologic findings in different organs to suggest a diagnosis and reconstruct the clinical course of the disease. Again, he would describe his observations and his thought process, thus teaching us gross pathology, analysis, and most interestingly the pathogenesis of the disease.

Although English was not his native language, Dr. Popper was a superb and effective lecturer. The secret to his success was based on his extensive and thorough preparation for every lecture well in advance. He selected all slides with extreme care, spent many hours in composing the text, and always asked for input from his colleagues, even in the selection of the different colors of his famous text slides. Clarity and organization were the keys to the success of his lectures. Due to his accent, medical students did not always understand what he said, but they certainly took home the important messages. In return for his efforts, Dr. Popper demanded an attentive and appreciative audience. We remember vividly that on one cold winter morning when Dr. Popper began his lecture, several of the sophomore students continued to chat or read *The New York Times*. Dr. Popper was furious, put on his coat, and started to walk out of the lecture hall, but the students dragged him back to the podium and then certainly paid attention. Often, Dr. Popper "tried out" his major lectures for international or national conferences on smaller groups, such as his residents or members of his research team. He taught and we learned; we asked questions and he learned.

Perhaps Dr. Popper's most effective and memorable teaching accomplishments were in small groups or on a one-to-one basis. His frequent and regular meetings with his fellows and members of the research group always remained a learning experience, even for the most experienced investigators. Dr. Popper's brilliant intellect was clearly evident when studies were designed or data were analyzed. Most of all, we enjoyed the Saturday afternoons when in a relaxed atmosphere devoid of the pressures of the work week, Dr. Popper would walk up and down in his office, puff on his pipe, and dictate crucial passages of a manuscript in preparation. He enjoyed our questions and challenges to his new ideas or hypotheses, we would argue, go back to the literature guided by his phenomenal memory for references, look at the slides again, and argue some more. By 6 p.m., we understood what he meant and he had crystallized his thoughts. It was then time to go home. He would pick up the telephone and call Lina, his wife: "Maidy, I'm coming home now."

Good-bye, Dr. Popper. Thank you. We will always miss you.

References

1. Popper H. A new curriculum. *Ann NY Acad Sci* 1965; 128:552–60.
2. Popper H. Current trends in curriculum redesign. *J Mt Sinai Hosp* 1968; 35:332–42.
3. Popper H. Currents in medical education in the United States. *J Mt Sinai Hosp* 1969; 36:348–60.
4. Popper H. The program at Mount Sinai School of Medicine and implications for teaching alcoholic liver disease. *Ann NY Acad Sci* 1971; 178:39–51.
5. Popper H, King DW. The situation of American Pathology 1975: education problems, yesterday, today and tomorrow. *Beitrage zur Pathologie* 1975; 156:85–94.
6. Popper H, Nosoff RM. Challenge to medical education in the United States. In: *In honor of Thomas Doxiadis*. Athens: Hospital "Evangelismos," 1976; 408–19.
7. Popper H. Our school of medicine. In the beginning. . . . *Mt Sinai Alumni Spectrum* 1977; 7:10–13.
8. Popper H. Die neuere Entwicklung der Medizin in den Vereinigten Staaten von Nordamerika. *Therapiewoche* 1977; 27:6540–8.

9. Popper H. Gustave L. Levy and the development of the medical school. *Mt Sinai J Med* 1977; 44:585–93.
10. Nosoff RM, Popper H. The current challenge to medical students in the United States. *Mt Sinai J Med* 1977; 44:602–12.
11. Popper H. MSSM: Ten years of basic sciences. *Mt Sinai Alumni Spectrum* 1978; 8:21–2.
12. Popper H. Tribute. In: *Sheila Sherlock: a career in medicine*. Welwyn Garden City, England: Smith Kline and French Laboratories, 1983.

14

Wolfgang Gerok, Freiburg

HANS POPPER, FREIBURG, AND HEPATOLOGY

Hans Popper's connections with Freiburg go back to the 1920s. In 1928, when he was a young assistant at the Institute of Pathology of the University of Vienna, he was invited to present a paper at the University Medical Clinic in Freiburg and then to stay on as guest of the university to study the processes of transudation in inflammatory conditions, using the methods he had developed for the determination of protein-bound carbohydrates. At that time, the University of Freiburg was a stronghold of medical–biological research: Franz Knoop, discoverer of the beta-oxidation of fatty acids and the processes of amino-acid degradation, was working in the field of biochemistry; Heinrich Wieland was working on the structure of cholesterol and bile acids at the Chemical Institute; Ludwig Aschoff, discoverer of the reticuloendothelial system, was head of the Institute of Pathology; studies of cholesterol metabolism were being carried out at the Department of Biochemistry of this institute by A. Schönheimer, and the head of the Institute of Biology was the development biologist, R. Spemann. Several of these research scientists were later awarded the Nobel Prize for their pioneering work.

Already during his first stay in Freiburg, as he often said later, Hans Popper was impressed not only by the scientific contact he enjoyed with other researchers, but also by the special character of the city of Freiburg itself. He came to love this city in the far southwest corner of Germany with its Gothic cathedral, its arcades and squares, which, with its proximity to France, Switzerland, and Italy, gave the city a southern European atmosphere and an air of openness. The Hans Popper perhaps also felt particularly at home in Freiburg because with its surroundings and its charm it reminded him of his Austrian homeland. In this region, the influence of Austria was, and still is, clearly evident, because after all it belonged to the Austrian Empire, as an Outer-Austrian patrimonial land, for more than 100 years.

In spite of the great problems and disappointments he experienced due to his forced emigration in 1938, Hans Popper quickly renewed contact with the research scientists in Germany and Austria after the end of the war. His first renewed contact with Freiburg and its university was his meeting with Ludwig Heilmeyer, then head of the University Medical Clinic in Freiburg, when they both received a doctorate from the Faculty of Medicine of Louvain in Belgium. Ludwig Heilmeyer introduced him to Dr. H. Falk, and it was together with him and Dr. Kurt Beck, then hepatologist at the Freiburg Clinic, that Hans Popper developed and realized the project for the International Freiburg Liver Symposia.

The first symposium, with the theme "Jaundice," was held in the autumn of 1967. The response in Germany and abroad was so overwhelming that these symposia are now held regularly, every 3 years, and have become an internationally recognized institution. Their aim is to give clinical hepatologists and representatives of related clinical disciplines and of the basic biomedical sciences an opportunity to meet and to provide practicing physicians with first-hand information on the latest developments and results in the field of hepatology. The main symposium, which is devoted to a general theme, was later flanked by satellite symposia on special subjects, so that finally there was a series of scientific symposia that became known as the "Freiburger Leberwoche"—the Freiburg Liver Week. The large number of participants and the limited hotel accommodations available in Freiburg eventually made it necessary to transfer this event to the nearby city of Basel in Switzerland. Very early, subjects were dealt with in the satellite symposia that today belong to the central working areas of hepatological research, for example collagen metabolism and fibrogenesis, bile-acid metabolism and biliary secretion, communications of liver cells, and regulation of genetic expression. With the choice of subjects and speakers, but above all with his contribution to the discussions and his legendary summaries of the results, Hans Popper left his decisive individual mark on these symposia. Always clearly in evidence was his great gift for building bridges between the different research results and between the different scientific disciplines and, on the basis of his immense knowledge, for developing original associations and fruitful hypotheses.

Hans Popper's delightful personality was always very much in evidence not only in the scientific parts of the Freiburg symposia but also in the social program. He loved the company of friends, the wine of the area around Freiburg, and the local atmosphere of the villages of the Black Forest or the wine districts of the Kaiserstuhl and the Markgräfler Land. When the local village bands were playing in their traditional costumes, and there was good wine on the table, Hans Popper was one of the happiest. It was then hardly possible to subdue his discourses, in his own special mixture of German and English, and his passion for dancing, especially with pretty young students. And it was also the enormous hospitality of Herbert Falk that made these gatherings such unforgettable occasions.

Hans Popper had many friends in the clinics and institutes of the Medical Faculty of Freiburg. On his regular visits to Europe, he very often came back to Freiburg in order to keep up to date with the latest research work and to discuss the results. Often on his arrival at Zurich Airport from the United States he would immediately go to a scientific conference at the clinic. There was no sign of jet lag when in the discussions he would take up and interpret the essentials of a scientific presentation. His knowledge, which he had stored in his brain, as if in a computer, and which he could recall on a key word at any time, enabled him to immediately recognize where interconnections existed to other directions of research. He was often able to interpret the results in a way that even the presenter himself had not recognized. In this, especially toward the younger research scientists, he never showed his superior knowledge and experience in an authoritarian way. His remarks in the discussions often began with an acknowledgment or a word of praise before immediately tackling the critical points and raising conceptual questions. Scientific conferences with Hans Popper were never boring but always stimulating and fascinating, due to his incisive ideas and his brilliant intellect.

Not least, I have to mention, in gratitude, that from the end of the war until the last year of his life Hans Popper gave positive help and encouragement to many young research scientists, not only at the University of Freiburg but also at many other German and Austrian universities. He would encourage them to persevere, in spite of the many frustrations, and to pursue an original hypothesis and direction of research and to look for new methods in order to find solutions for difficult scientific problems. But as the "reigning monarch of hepatology" and as the scientific world citizen he had become, he also opened the doors of the research institutes of the United States to European research scientists after the war. One of his most important concerns, to which he devoted enormous energy and enthusiasm up to the last year of his life, was to discover new talented young scientists who were pursuing original ideas and to help them develop. Many members of the Freiburg Medical Faculty, and especially of the University Medical Clinic, have experienced and benefitted from his unselfish and generous help and encouragement, always given with his inimitable Viennese charm.

Unforgettable for us is the award to Hans Popper of the honorary doctorate from the Medical Faculty of the University of Freiburg. To receive such an honor was an enormous satisfaction to him, and he was unable to conceal his great pleasure and pride. After the award ceremony and his presentation, "Hepatitis-B Infection and Liver-Cell Carcinoma," he was joined by his friends at a well-known historic hostelry in the Black Forest. Rarely had I seen Hans Popper so proud and happy, so amusing and fascinating as then, as he recounted the chances and decisions, the encounters and the experiences of his long life. The wheel had turned the full circle: here, where 60 years earlier he had been invited, as a young scientist, for a working visit, he was now being honored as a research scientist of international repute. We were honoring a world citizen in whom the spiritual currents of the Old World and the New World were joined, an original and versatile research scientist, and, last but not least, a good and extremely dependable friend.

15

Helmut Greim, Neuherberg

"LEBERRABBI"

From May 1970 to May 1973, I worked as visiting research associate professor of pathology with Hans Popper at Mount Sinai. I first met him shortly after my arrival in New York. My first impression was that I would never be able to understand him, despite the fact that in my home institute, Herbert Remmer's Institute of Toxicology in Tuebingen, we had many English-speaking visitors, which provided us with some experience in that language. However, possibly due to my family's Austrian-Bavarian vernacular, I increasingly became used to his way of speaking English. In addition to my own problems, it was clear that Hans also met with difficulties when communicating in English. Once he returned from a Senate hearing in Washington and told us of the following distressing experience: One of the senators asked him a question, which Hans did not understand. He asked the senator to repeat the question, but was again unable to decipher its meaning. In response to his request that the senator repeat the question again, the senator resorted to asking the question in German.

Hans, however, admitted that, in general, native Americans were quite tolerant of those who acquired English in school and continued to learn English during their stay in the United States. He warned us, however, that when you arrive in the United States everyone praises your good English. After 5 years, they assure you that your English is not bad. Thus, it is quite deflating when your own children tell you that you will never be able to learn the language. Keeping this in mind, he always asked us to prepare both an introductory and a summarizing slide when giving a lecture in English. He said, "Your audience may have problems with your accent. At best, they will become used to it. Beware, however, that, at worst, they might not be able to understand a word. These two slides will insure that at least they will get the message of your presentation." Fenton Schaffner was our English expert. Hans always accepted Schaffner's advice on English as definitive when the English in our manuscripts, including Hans' own, was questioned.

Questions on English usage often came up at the "Monday night meetings." The general purpose of these meetings, however, was to discuss ongoing research, manuscripts in preparation, and future research activities. In addition, many of Mount Sinai's political problems were discussed. To the foreigners in our group, these discussions helped us to understand research politics and organizational problems involved in running a large medical school in the United States. Although many of the problems were familiar to us, they tended to be slightly altered by national differences. Occasionally, governmental pressure seemed to decide university policies. For example, Popper said tongue-in-cheek that the optimal characteristics for achieving entrance to The Mount Sinai School of Medicine were that you were black, female, and Jewish.

Several basic principles were introduced into our attitude regarding the publication of manuscripts.

1. Publish whatever interesting and relevant data you have. Do not leave them in the drawer or else all the money spent for these experiments will have been wasted.

2. Never submit a manuscript in which the data and the ideas are not presented in the best possible language. Hans indicated that he himself at least had learned that in Klippschule (grammar school). Occasionally, Hans, when unhappy with our manuscripts, even questioned whether we had ever attended the Klippschule.

3. After completion of a manuscript, keep it in a drawer for 2 weeks, then read it again and correct those errors you made during the hectic time of initial preparation. However, you had better not delay delivering a completed paper to Hans when he was interested in early publication, which was usually the case. On one occasion, after a manuscript had been discussed, rewritten, and, I thought, finalized, I left for a holiday trip to Florida after asking for permission. At the next Monday night meeting, Hans expressed dissatisfaction that I did not come up with the final, polished paper. The word dissatisfaction is mild considering his actual response to my absence. Frank Hutterer quickly got to me by telephone, and my holiday in Florida came to a premature ending.

4. The reviewer is always right. Unfortunately, his comments are predict-

able, and it is only because of our sloppy thinking that we did not identify the false statements or misconceptions in the manuscripts ourselves prior to their submission.

5. Always send the manuscript to the journal with the best reputation in the special research area of your paper. There are others of slightly less distinction that might be honored with the manuscript in the event that the initial reviewers were blind to its great value and relevance to modern biology.

Since completing my medical training and passing my examinations I had devoted my career exclusively to biochemical pharmacology. One of the great benefits of my stay with Hans was to consider the practical consequences of our experimental findings. Most of our experimental work in those days was the investigation of mechanisms of intrahepatic cholestasis. To see how the results of our work could be applied to the practical aspects of human hepatology, we frequently attended the "slide conferences" of the Pathology Department. Hans refused to be told the anamnesis or diagnosis of the cases before considering the slides. Instead, he used to discuss all of the major and minor pathological changes on the slide, usually a liver biopsy or postmortem sample, which was projected on the screen. Despite the fact that Hans often disagreed with the attending physician, who had, in fact, correctly diagnosed the case, it was fascinating to observe him apply his tremendous wealth of knowledge and experience to speculate on the underlying disease.

It was great to work with him at Mount Sinai, and his visits to my institute in Munich taught my co-workers why I was so fascinated with his scientific personality. Despite his superior knowledge of the liver, he refused to be called the "Leberpapst." Perhaps we should give him the posthumous title that he proposed instead, namely, "Leberrabbi."

16

Pauline Hall, Bedford Park

As an aspiring hepatopathologist, I read many of Hans Popper's numerous publications on the liver, both those that appeared during my time as a trainee in the 1960s and 1970s as well as many of the earlier classic papers. I remember feeling overawed to be in the presence of such a great man when I attended my first Basel Liver Week in 1979. I was amazed on actually meeting him to discover that he knew of the halothane hepatitis research work being done by the small group led by Professor Michael Cousins, director of Anaesthesia and Intensive Care, Flinders Medical Centre, South Australia.

My friendship with Hans Popper began in Basel. Undoubtedly, it was our shared interest in halothane hepatoxicity that brought us together, but over the years we became very good friends and got to know each other's families. Hans and Lina helped me through several crises in my personal life and encouraged me to "find solace" in my work.

HALOTHANE HEPATITIS   I hope it is appropriate to give a little background information about this topic, which in the 1960s and 1970s was highly controversial. The debate for and against the role of halothane in fulminant hepatitic necrosis was passionately contested by many anesthetists, clinicians, and pathologists in the United States.

Halothane was introduced as an inhalational anesthetic agent in 1956 and rapidly gained acceptance because it was nonexplosive, noninflammable, and could be delivered in precise doses. However, by 1958, case reports of fatal liver injury following halothane anesthesia began to appear. The relatively low incidence (1:10,000–1:36,000) of severe and usually fatal liver injury together with the nonspecific nature of the hepatic injury confounded the problem. Hans Popper and many other eminent members of the medical profession were involved in the National Halothane Study, which exonerated halothane as a hepatotoxin (1). The subsequent recognition of the hepatotoxicity of halothane must have been one of the rare instances when Hans Popper had to reverse an opinion. The manner in which he was prepared to publicly admit to an error in judgment should be an example to everyone in our profession. Hans maintained a passionate interest in the pathogenesis of halothane hepatotoxicity and closely monitored the work of research groups around the world. He visited many of the groups, including our South Australian group; we supplied him with preprints of our papers and gladly accepted both his praise and his criticism.

Hans was particularly interested in the guinea pig model for halothane hepatotoxicity that was developed by Christine Lunam, one of my higher degree students (2). Whenever I was in the United States, I would visit Hans at Mount Sinai Hospital to show him histological sections of our most recent experiments. He was excited by sections of the injured guinea pig liver and thought that the delayed appearance of the lesion together with the prominent lymphocytic infiltrate indicated an immunologically mediated injury.

Michael Cousins and I plan to write a monograph on halothane hepatitis once the controversy over the pathogenesis of the liver injury—direct toxicity versus immunologically mediated injury—has been resolved. I would like to record the sincere thanks of all the members of our halothane research group to Hans Popper for his enthusiastic support, encouragement, and valued criticisms of our work and to announce in advance our wish to dedicate our monograph to him.

HANS AND LINA POPPER IN AUSTRALIA, 1980   Hans and Lina visited Australia and New Zealand during February and March 1980. As usual, this was a working holiday for Hans. Hans and I were invited to contribute to a session on halothane hepatitis at the Asian Pacific Association for the Study of Liver Meeting in Auckland, New Zealand. The Poppers then visited Brisbane; Lawrie Powell describes this visit in her contribution to this book. However, I thought it would be a good idea to ask Lina for her account of the remarkable events that occurred during their brief visit to the barrier reef resort, Heron Island. With Lina's permission, I have included the following extract from a recent letter.

> At my insistence and contrary to Hans' wishes (I won sometimes) we were to spend a few days on Heron Island between Brisbane and Melbourne where he was to give a named lecture early Monday morning. We were to leave the island Sunday afternoon on one of those small four-seater helicopters to Gladstone and go on to Melbourne from there. We had a great time until Sunday morning when we woke to the announcement that a cyclone was on its way and nobody knew how long the planes could fly people off the island. Hans, who was very compulsive and conscientious about his

professional obligations, was very tense and almost panicky. We talked to the people in the office and they promised to do their best. They indeed flew him out on the last helicopter. There was only one seat and I insisted he take it. They promised him that I would be on the next flight. I was: Wednesday at 10 a.m. There was no communication between the mainland and the island and neither of us knew what happened to the other for 3 days. We met again in Sydney.

We both enjoyed the trip tremendously: so different, new impressions, gorgeous nature, new people, and professional contacts and stimulation and on top *adventure*.

Hans Popper's visit to Sydney was sponsored by the Royal Australian College of Physicians. Hans, together with Prof. Michael Cousins, director of Anaesthesia and Intensive Care, FMC, South Australia, and Prof. Leo Strunin, head of Anaesthesiology, Foothills Hospital, Calgary, Canada, who was sponsored by the Royal College of Physicians and Surgeons, Canada, took part in a unique Australian meeting on halothane hepatitis, which was organized jointly by the Royal Australasian College of Surgeons and the Royal Australasian College of Physicians. Michael Cousins was pleased to find himself "on the same side" as Hans, while Leo Strunin remained more skeptical of the toxicity of halothane.

Hans had not recovered from the emotional trauma of "losing his Lina" by the time he reached Adelaide—the story of the cyclone dominated his conversation for many days and no doubt has been retold many times. Lina, as usual, provided Hans with constant comfort and reassurance and I think they were able to enjoy their few days in South Australia.

Hans spent a generous amount of time with the halothane research group at Flinders Medical Centre; our higher degree students were delighted to have the opportunity to discuss their work with him. We had recently completed an interesting study on "genetic differences" in reductive metabolism and hepatotoxicity of halothane in three rat strains; we appreciated the help he gave us with the final stages of the manuscript (3).

The Flinders University medical students attended Hans' memorable lecture, "The Pathogenesis of Alcoholic Liver Disease." They were amazed by his complex multicolored slides, which he used to compensate for his accent, which many people found difficult to understand.

I recall that our social activities in Adelaide were also highly memorable. My close friend and colleague Associate Professor Malcolm Mackinnon and his wife Allison and my husband and I took Hans and Lina to lunch under the vines at The Barn, a restaurant cum art gallery in the Southern Vales. After lunch, we tasted wines in several nearby wineries; Ingoldbys and Piramimima are the ones I remember. Hans, like most of our overseas visitors, was unprepared for the excellence of South Australian wines. We then had afternoon tea with my mother-in-law, who lived nearby. By the time we arrived, Hans was both lively and loquacious; he roamed about the house "holding forth," as my husband described it, on a wide variety of topics, none of which can be recalled by either of us. My mother-in-law, an elderly lady of "delicate sensibilities" had never met such an extraordinary extrovert; nevertheless, once she and Hans found they had a shared interest in the history of the German migration to the Barossa Valley (another excellent wine-growing district) she responded warmly to him and later admitted how much she had enjoyed their conversation.

We also had a small dinner party at Horsts, one of Adelaide's trendy restaurants. I remember Hans dancing with all of the pretty young women—the restaurant did not have a dance floor so Hans danced around the bar and between the tables!

Michael Cousins subsequently wrote to Hans inviting him to spend a "sabbatical" in Australia. The invitation was declined graciously; Hans had declared that, after the trauma of "losing Lina," his first trip to Australia would definitely also be his last.

Hans encouraged me to send abstracts of our halothane work to the 1980 IASL/APASL meetings. The photo of Hans with Lina and I (see Fig. 14 in photo section) was taken just after I had presented one of my papers. Hans then took us out for a leisurely lunch. By this time, Hans had several health problems, which he hated to admit. We had taken far too long over lunch and had to walk briskly back to the meeting—Hans became short of breath but refused to slacken his pace—as always his commitment to hepatology took priority over personal inconveniences including illness.

"ALCOHOLIC LIVER DISEASE"   I had already formulated an outline for my book on alcoholic liver disease by the time I met Hans in 1979. I thought that, if I had sufficient epidemiological information about the disease in various countries, I might gain insight into risk factors for alcohol-associated liver injury. My observations had convinced me that the liver injury was not simply a dose-related effect. Hans offered me invaluable help with the book, although he thought my search for risk factors via epidemiological studies would probably be unrewarding. In my preface, I said that I would like the book to be my personal tribute to Hans Popper in conjunction with his 80th birthday celebrations.

Hans wrote the foreword to this book—it truly was an amazing piece of work. He wrote it as a draft long before I had received chapters from many of the contributors. The foreword needed very little changing when the book was in its final stages. Almost 10 years later, his comments remain valid, and most of the questions he raised remain unanswered, as will be apparent from the following extracts.

Alcoholic liver disease therefore represents not only a major medical, social, and psychological problem, but can also be looked upon as a model of human disease with one well-recognized initiating factor but modulated by others. This in turn permits the evaluation in man, of the role of other factors responsible or contributing to alcoholic liver disease.

Many riddles persist even in the pathobiology of alcoholic liver disease. The mechanism of the initial fat accumulation in the liver is the best understood. Far more mysterious is the pathogenesis of alcoholic hepatitis, so far not effectively reproduced in experimental animals. The mechanism of hepatocellular necrosis is not established in either alcoholic liver injury, or in many other types of liver disease. The pathogenesis of alcoholic cirrhosis still requires clarification. The possibility that cirrhosis may develop without a significant hepatitic precursor stage has to be excluded. Even more problematic is the pathogenesis of hepatocellular carcinoma in alcoholics, not necessarily associated with cirrhosis.

In introducing this volume, one may hope that a scholarly review of the state of the art will contribute to the solution of some of the unresolved problems. Moreover, the spread of information is a powerful tool by itself in the management of a disease, particularly when it is potentially preventable. However, in stressing prevention in this introduction, one should keep in mind that the production of wine from grapes is one of the oldest horticultural achievements of mankind and was already ancient when the Greeks enjoyed their wine. It is also a fact that many of the contributors to this volume, including myself, still believe that moderate drinking may add to the enjoyment of their lives.

Over the years, Hans, Lina, and I exchanged numerous letters and several small gifts, among them a book and a silk scarf, which I particularly treasure. I am very proud of the artwork on the front cover of the alcohol book, since it was done by my youngest son, Ross. Following publication of the book, Hans Popper was the only person who wrote specifically to comment on its appearance.

1st February, 1985

Dear Pauline:

I just received your handsome book on *Alcoholic Liver Disease*. It has been brought out very elegantly and I want to congratulate you on an excellent job. I hope it will have the success which it deserves.

I hope everything is all right with you. Lina and I send you our best wishes and I hope to see you soon.

Very sincerely yours,

Hans Popper, M.D.

These selected recollections have been predominantly about Hans, with little mention of Lina Popper. As all their friends know, Lina was always at his side (cyclones permitting) to love and comfort him as well as to take care of the practical aspects of his life. It was Lina's total devotion to all his needs that enabled Hans to fully utilize his exceptional skills. Even if the world of hepatology could produce another Hans Popper I doubt if there would be a Lina to ease his way.

References

1. Bunker JP, Forrest WH, Mostellar F, Vandam LD, eds. *The national halothane study*. Bethesda: National Institutes of Health, National Institute of General Medical Sciences, 1969.
2. Lunam CA, Cousins MJ, Hall P de la M. A guinea pig model of halothane-associated hepatotoxicity in the absence of enzyme induction and hypoxia. *Pharmacol Exp Ther* 1985; 232:802–09.
3. Gourlay GK, Adams JF, Cousins MJ, Hall P. Genetic differences in reductive metabolism and hepatotoxicity of halothane in three rat strains. *Anaesthesiology* 1981; 55:96–103.
4. Hall P, ed. *Alcoholic liver disease: pathobiology, epidemiology and clinical features*. London: Edward Arnold, 1985.

17

Sarah C. Kalser, Bethesda

In 1975, Dr. Popper served on the prestigious Advisory Council of the National Institute of Arthritis, Metabolism and Diabetes [now the National Institute of Diabetes and Digestive and Kidney Diseases (NIDDK)]. As a member of that body, which reviews all research grant applications and recommends to the director those that they judge to be worthy of support, Dr. Popper was well aware of the many bright, promising young investigators whose applications could not be accepted because of limited funds. Parenthetically, these earlier days now look like the good old days compared with the current climate in which even fewer investigators can be paid. This climate of discouragement for productive investigators and for promising new investigators troubled him deeply. At the time, he himself held an Institute grant and had been an Institute grantee for 15 years. With all his energy, insights, and sound basic and clinical expertise, he could have continued his supported research for nearly another 15 years of his investigative career. However, he made a decision at that point, which I have not seen made by any other investigator I have known in my 20 years as a research grants administrator of the liver and biliary diseases program at NIDDK. He decided to voluntarily terminate his NIDDK support; not because he was moving into a new position such as sometimes happens when investigators go to work for industry or give up research for a private clinical practice. No, Dr. Popper decided to give up his research grant because he said it was more important that some young investigator receive that support. He said he could still do his research by helping other investigators, reading his own slides, stimulating ideas in the community, etc. You know the rest of the story. Dr. Hans Popper probably published more scholarly papers, stimulated more scholarly research, received more honorary degrees and traveled to more foreign shores to promulgate liver research in the last 15 years of his life than during his years as an NIH-supported investigator. Instead of the termination of his grant terminating his productivity, the termination of his grant freed him to do more imaginative research, learn molecular biology, and to devote his great energies to stimulate investigators and investigations throughout the United States and the world.

18

Donald King, Chicago

In 1975, a dinner was held at a club in New York City to celebrate three outstanding pathologists in the New York area: Hans Popper, Harry Zimmerman, and Hirum Houston Merritt. At that time, I considered it an "around retirement time recognition ceremony." As the years passed, it finally emerged as a minor mid-career honor. Hans Popper's persistent drive to continue to do everything well and not give an inch to physical, mental, or emotional stresses of age, was the single most obvious and most admired trait of this extraordinary man it was my privilege to know for over 30 years.

One might fill pages with anecdotes relating to his intensity, his energy, and his intellect. His rare grasp of the entire field of medicine from the molecular biology of collagen, bile metabolism, the delta factor to the clinical signs and symptoms of chronic active hepatitis continually reflected the breadth as well as the depth of his knowledge.

This tribute will not reiterate his contributions to The Mount Sinai Medical Center or Cook County Hospital, to pathology societies in the county, state, and nation, or to personal contacts, which led to significant state and national legislation. Although many people claim credit for the NIH section on digestive diseases, his meeting at a pathology seminar at Arden House with Paul Rogers, then Chairman of the House Committee on Health, did the legislation no harm. This essay does take note but will not testify extensively to his voluminous bibliography including lectures, articles, monographs, chapters, and many books for which he was contributor, editor, and original author. More important are the tutorials he conducted on science, medicine, ethics, politics, and history with me personally and literally and figuratively with hundreds of others of his colleagues.

Hans continued this fearless, seldom fearsome, moving, restless pattern through his 70s and 80s. He never believed in allowing age to interfere in any manner with his travels, his writing, his lectures, and his full participation in the life of his family, university, and community.

As one gets older, one appreciates the characteristics of the true physician epitomized by Robert Louis Stevenson (in *Underwoods*, Dedication).

> There are men and classes of men that stand above the common herd: the soldier, the sailor, and the shepherd not unfrequently; the artist rarely; rarelier still, the clergyman; the physician almost as a rule. He is the flow [such as it is] of our civilization. . . . Generosity he has, such as is possible to those who practice an art, never to those who drive a trade; discretion, tested by a hundred secrets; tact; tried in a thousand embarrassments; and what are more important, Heraclean cheerfulness and courage.

One rarely hears this accolade reported anymore, although Charles Huggins used to quote it at dinners held for people he particularly respected, at the University of Chicago. The profession has grown from an elite group of a few thousand to several hundred thousand practitioners, scientists, and administrators. It has become super specialized and changed its personnel base from individual caring with duty, responsibility, and curiosity to molecular biology and large societal, socioeconomic, and ethical issues.

It is difficult to believe that Huntington only described one disease and only wrote one paper and that Bright wrote very few papers, since both contributed so significantly to medicine. Despite Hans' acute awareness of molecular biology, he often remarked that his most important scientific instrument was his microscope.

The government now intrudes on every level. The young not only justly question the complexity and injustices of the system, but attack remorselessly with few constructive alternatives. The business sense of the medical profession is high; 600 billion dollars a year with homes, cars, planes, fine food, administration, and too many patients and too little time to read, walk, listen to Mahler, or reflect.

The pace is even more frantic as time passes with little compassion for those who fall by the wayside. Hans Popper did not fall by the wayside, but, as the epitome of a true physician, scholar, and gentleman, he respected and protected those who slowed the pace. For this alone his friends will always remember him with great appreciation.

19

Sherman Kupfer, New York

It is now 34 years since I heard Hans Popper's name spoken for the first time. I had come to Mount Sinai as an intern in July 1948. In 1955, I was appointed research assistant in medicine at The Mount Sinai Hospital, and along with research and clinical teaching duties, I served as staff to the Research Administrative Committee (RAC). This committee was the forerunner to what is now known almost everywhere as the IRB, the Institutional Review Board, which must approve all research involving human subjects. At Mount Sinai, RAC had been functioning since 1937, long before review of research was to be mandated by the federal government. In 1955, Dr. Alexander B. Gutman, then director of the Department of Medicine, was the senior professional member of the committee. George Lee, a vice-president of the board of trustees, served as committee chairman at its monthly meetings.

In 1956, while serving in my role as staff to this committee, Dr. Gutman told me that Hans Popper was being considered as a possible successor to Dr. Paul Klemperer. Dr. Klemperer had long since earned his reputation as a living legend. It was not going to be easy to find his successor.

Drs. Gutman and Steinberg (the latter was director of The Mount Sinai Hospital) and, on another occasion, Joseph Klingenstein (president of the board of trustees) visited Dr. Popper in Chicago and tried to persuade him to accept the position as director of pathology at The Mount Sinai Hospital. After considerable hesitation, Dr. Popper did agree to serve in this capacity starting in 1957.

Dr. Popper already was well on his way to becoming "Mr. Liver," so to speak. But these details have been better delegated to others. However, Dr. Popper's name was not unknown to me when first mentioned in 1956. That name rang a bell in a context other than the liver. Those who wanted to be identified as being knowledgeable in renal physiology had, at one time or another, read Homer Smith's classic treatise entitled *The Kidney* (1). Dr. Smith had listed seven papers in which "Popper, H." appeared.

In my opinion, one of the most important contributions was that which described the use of the plasma creatinine concentration as an index of renal function. The widespread and continuing use of the endogenous creatinine clearance as a quantitative measure of renal function and index of glomerular filtration rate is based on this work. I do not believe that many of my colleagues in nephrology are aware that this was one of Dr. Popper's many contributions to renal physiology and renal histology (2–16). Dr. Popper had a substantial background in biochemistry, and he made very respectable contributions in this field. This training and expertise was an important component to his observations on and contributions to renal function. In 1940, he was invited to lecture at a symposium on vitamins held at The Mount Sinai Hospital. His talk was on the body distribution of vitamin A. This lecture was reported in the *Journal of The Mount Sinai Hospital* (17).

My first meeting with Dr. Popper was shortly after his arrival at Mount Sinai in 1957. My assigned task was to introduce him to the workings of RAC, of which he was to become a member, and ultimately the senior member of its professional group. That meeting was an experience with a capital E. It was clear that Dr. Popper had made the transition to Mount Sinai as if he had never been anywhere else. During our first conversation, Dr. Popper expressed to me his interest in being known as a clinician and, in particular, a gastroenterologist. I was gently, but firmly, informed that he would be delighted to speak at medical grand rounds in that capacity. It was at this point that I asked him if he was the H. Popper referred to in Dr. Smith's book, *The Kidney*. There was a prolonged, almost frightening pause, something most unusual for the Dr. Popper I would come to know so well. He even may have bitten off the stem of his pipe, but I do not know that for sure. Then he smiled broadly, stood up, and came over to clap me on the shoulder. "Who are you, Kupfer (using the German pronunciation of my name which he always did), that you would know anything about my work on the kidney?" He went on to elaborate on kidney physiology and kidney pathology. He obviously relished the opportunity. There was no question that he was an expert on the kidney. His secretary finally knocked on the door and interrupted our meeting to say that his next appointment already had been waiting for sometime. We never had gotten to the supposed topic of our meeting, RAC. But it was clear to me that Dr. Popper was going to be a giant at Mount Sinai in his own time.

The question of having a School of Medicine at Mount Sinai had been raised on very few previous occasions. In 1960, Dr. Popper became head of the professional group of RAC. William T. Golden, a member of the board of trustees, already had begun his service as chairman of RAC. At one of his first meetings with the committee, Mr. Golden suggested that an outside group of experts be invited to review the hospital's ongoing research efforts. This suggestion was not met with much enthusiasm from the professional staff, except for Drs. Popper and Gutman. At a subsequent separate meeting of the professional members of the committee, Dr. Gutman reiterated his view that any outside review of research at Mount Sinai would be given high marks. Dr. Popper stated that he agreed with Dr. Gutman, and that this was a great opportunity to initiate a discussion for creating a new medical school at Mount Sinai. He was positive that such a discussion, in conjunction with what he too felt would be a highly favorable outcome to the research review, would culminate in a decision by the board of trustees to proceed with the creation of a new medical school. This argument persuaded the professional group to endorse the review. Shortly thereafter, RAC recommended to the board of trustees that an outside review of the Hospital's research program be undertaken. In 1961, three eminent consultants, Drs. William B. Castle, W. Barry Wood, and Walter Bauer, were duly appointed to visit the hospital, to conduct the review, and to render a report on the quality of its current research program. Dr. Bauer was unable to attend the sessions.

I was given the task of organizing the meetings, which set the final agenda of the review and some of the rehearsals. I vividly recall the long agenda, and the many outstanding presentations that were made by the professional staff, particularly the research fellows and junior staff, some of whom are now senior members of the faculty. Suffice it to say, Dr. Popper, in particular, was thrilled with how the review had been organized, with the scientific content of the presentations, and with the crisp manner in which they were delivered. He was sure that Drs. Castle and Wood were extremely favorably impressed by the research presentations and that their report would stress the trustees' responsibility for promoting a leading role for Mount Sinai in medical research and education. The report did exactly that. Dr. Popper told me that the consultants had stated that such a role only could be met by Mount Sinai having its own School of Medicine. Moreover, they were reported to have said that the current group of highly qualified staff and those who might be recruited in the future would best be retained in a medical school setting. In my opinion, it was Dr. Popper's vision and drive, a force not to be dismissed, that made it impossible for the trustees to come to any other decision. He was instrumental in pressing for immediate action. With the election of Gustave L. Levy as president of the board of trustees in 1962, planning to create a new School of Medicine began in earnest.

Dr. Popper was in truth the father of the School of Medicine and its first leader, even though Dr. George James was named to serve as the school's first dean in 1965. Dr. Popper became dean with Dr. James' untimely death in 1972.

It was a great privilege to have served with Dr. Popper at the very conception of The Mount Sinai School of Medicine. Dr. Popper's academic accomplishments, and his contributions to renal physiology and pathology, and to medical education (17–23) made him more than just "Mr. Liver," a title in and of itself so richly deserved. To me, these contributions everlastingly assure him of being remembered as a "giant among giants."

References

1. Smith HW. *The kidney. Structure and function in health and disease*. New York: Oxford Medical Publications, 1950.
2. Popper H, Mandel E, Mayer H. Schnellmethode zur Beurteilung der Urämic als Ersatz der Reststickstoffbestimmung. *Klin Wochenschr* 1937; 16:987.
3. Popper H, Mandel E, Mayer H. Zur Kreatininbestimmung in Blute. *Biochem Z* 1937;291:394.
4. Fuchs F, Popper H. Über die Gewehsspalten der Niere. *Virchows Arch Pathol Anat* 1937; 299:203.
5. Popper H, Mandel E, Mayer H. Über die diagnostiche Bedeutung der Plasmakreatininbestimmung. *Z Klin Med* 1937; 133:56.
6. Popper H. Glomerulusinsuffizienz and tubuläre Funktiensstörung. *Klin Wochenschr* 1937; 16:1454.
7. Fuchs F, Popper H. Die Wasserverschiebung im Nierenmark. *Klin Wochenschr* 1937; 16:1708.
8. Popper H, Mandel E. Filtrations—und Resorptionsleistung in der Nierenpathologie. *Ergeb Inn Med Kinderheilkd* 1937; 53:685.
9. Fuchs F, Popper H. Blut und Saftströmung in der Niere (zur klinischen Bedeutung des Niereninterstitiums). *Ergeb Inn Med Kinderheilkd* 1938; 54:1.
10. Popper H, Brod J. Die physiologischen Schwankungen der Nierenarbeit. *Z Klin Med* 1938; 134:196.
11. Arkin A, Popper H. Urea resorption and relation between creatinine and urea clearance in renal disease. *Arch Intern Med* 1940; 65:626.
12. Gruenwald P, Popper H. The histogenesis and physiology of the renal glomerulus in early postnatal life. *J Urol* 1940; 43:452.
13. Kozoll DD, Steigmann F, Popper H. Studies of pectin administration to patients not in shock. *Proc Soc Exp Biol Med* 1943; 53:66.
14. Popper H, Loeffler E. Fluorescent granules at the glomerular pole of human kidneys. *Proc Soc Exp Biol Med* 1943; 53:68.
15. Popper H, Volk BW, Meyer KA, Kozoll DD, Steigmann F. Evaluation of gelatin and pectin solutions as substitutes for plasma in the treatment of shock. Histologic changes produced in human beings. *Arch Surg* 1945; 50:34.
16. Popper H, Steigmann F, Dyniewicz HA. Plasma vitamin A level in renal disease. *Am J Clin Pathol* 1945; 15:272.
17. Popper H. The distribution of vitamin A in the body. *J Mt Sinai Hosp* 1940: 7:119.
18. Popper H. New objectives in medical education. *Ann NY Acad Sci* 1965; 128:478.
19. Popper H. A new curriculum. *Ann NY Acad Sci* 1965; 128:552.
20. Popper H. The Mount Sinai concept. *Clin Res* 1965; 13:500.
21. Popper H, Koffler D. The goal. *J Mt Sinai Hosp* 1967; 34:401.
22. Popper H. Mt. Sinai: how a hospital builds a medical school. *Science* 1967; 158:614.
23. Popper H. A hospital as the basis of a new medical school. *J Med Educ* 1970; 45:571.

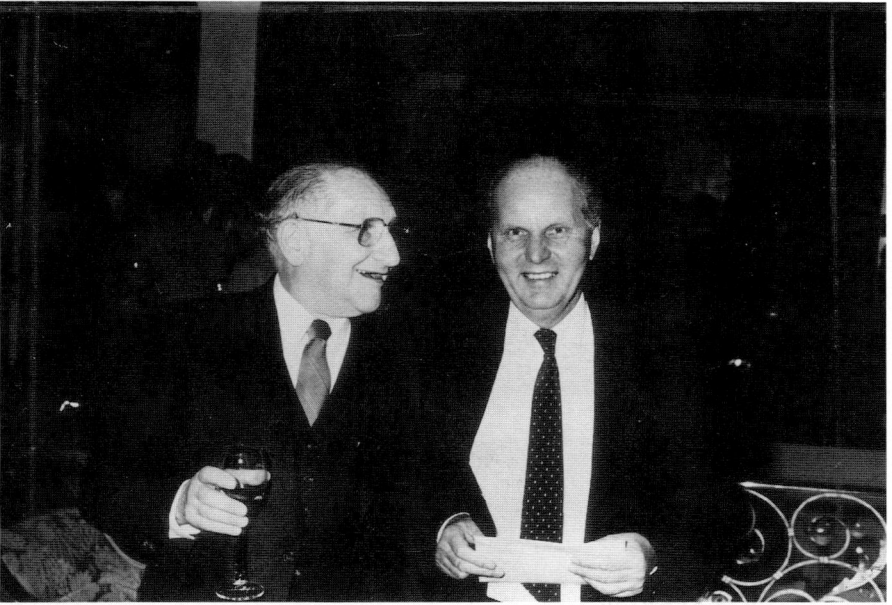

FIG. 1. Fruitful and sometimes mysterious discussions between Hans Popper, the brilliant scientist with a lot of sense for business, and Herbert Falk, a splendid businessman with a lot of sense for science. *(Courtesy of Leonardo Bianchi.)*

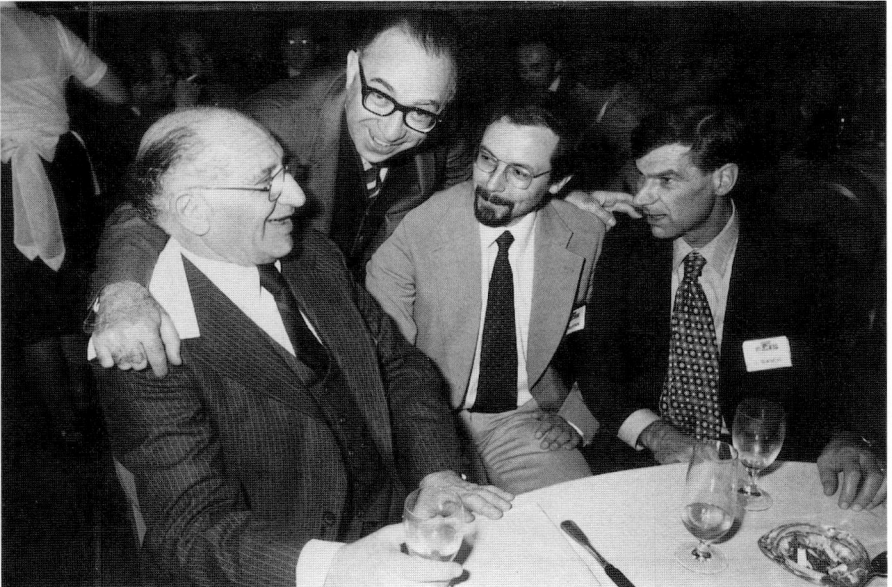

FIG. 2. "Let us conceive the liver cell membrane as a flow machine. . . ." Relaxation after a meeting day. From left to right: Hans Popper, Emmanuel Farber (Toronto), Werner Reutter (Berlin), and Piccio Bianchi (Basel). *(Courtesy of Leonardo Bianchi and Herbert Falk.)*

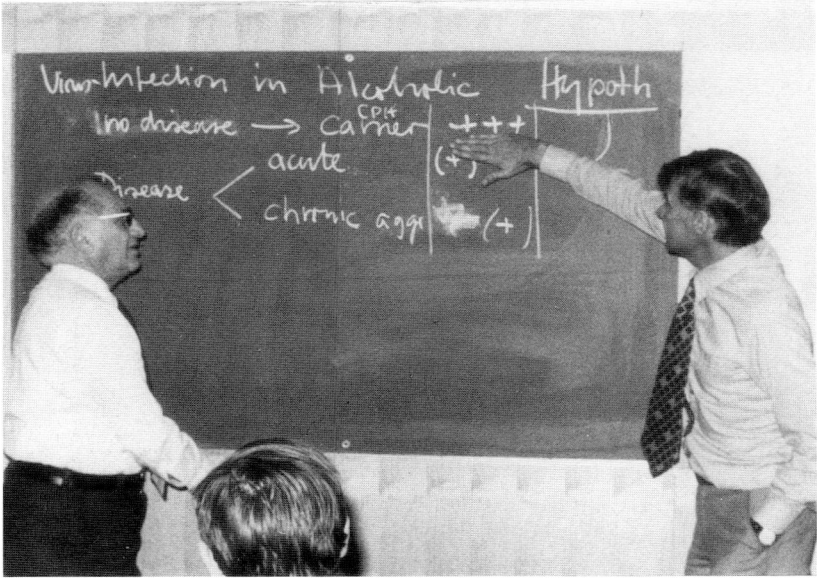

FIG. 3. Discussion at the blackboard, Zurich, 1978 during the planning of the 1979 Basel Liver Week. *(Courtesy of Leonardo Bianchi and Peter Scheuer.)*

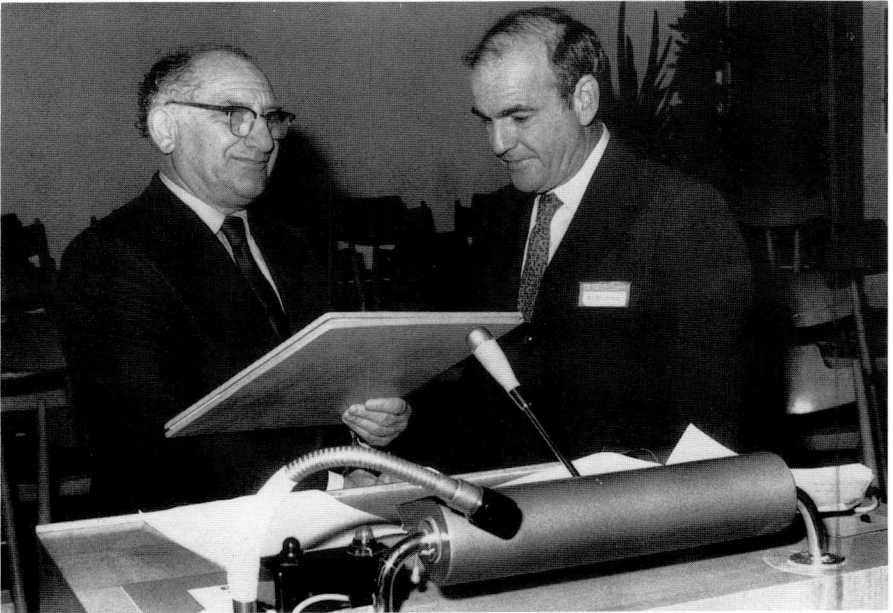

FIG. 4. Hans Popper and Baruch S. Blumberg in Freiburg, October 1973.
(Courtesy of Baruch S. Blumberg.)

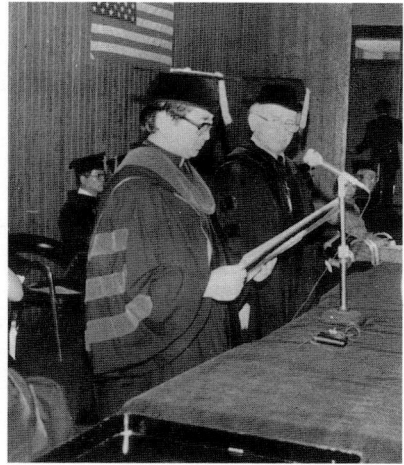

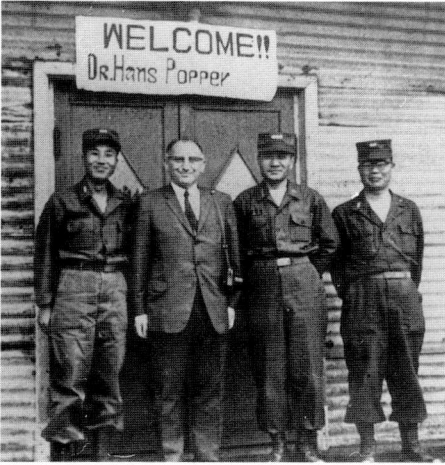

FIG. 5. (**Left**) Dr. Popper visited the 63rd ROK Army Hospital, Taejon, Korea, in June 1961 as a U.S. Army consultant. He was photographed with Col. S. N. Kim. *(Courtesy of Whan Kook Chung.)*

FIG. 6. (**Right**) Catholic University Medical College in Seoul conferred on Dr. Popper the degree of honorary Doctor of Medicine (July 1978). *(Courtesy of Whan Kook Chung.)*

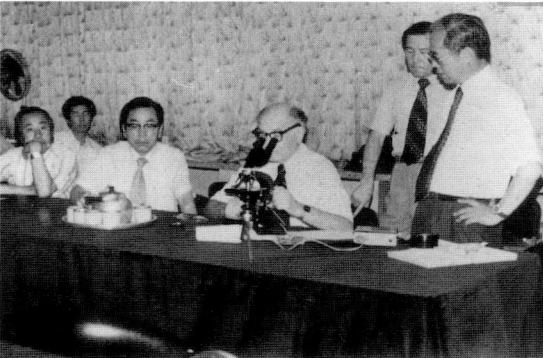

FIG. 7. Liver biopsy slide conference held at the Catholic University Medical College at Seoul (July 6, 1978).
(Courtesy of Whan Kook Chung.)

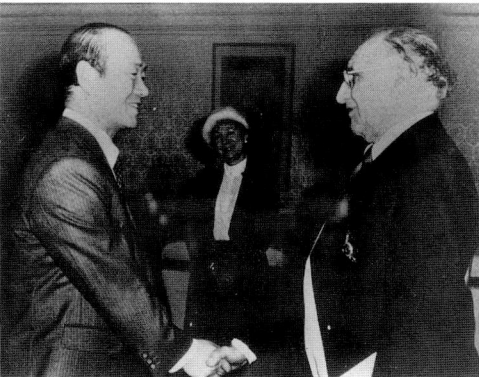

FIG. 8. Professor Popper, who was the initiator of the "Seoul International Liver Symposium," shakes hands with President Chun Doo Whan after being awarded the Order of Mugungwha (February 1982). Mrs. Popper looks on.
(Courtesy of Whan Kook Chung.)

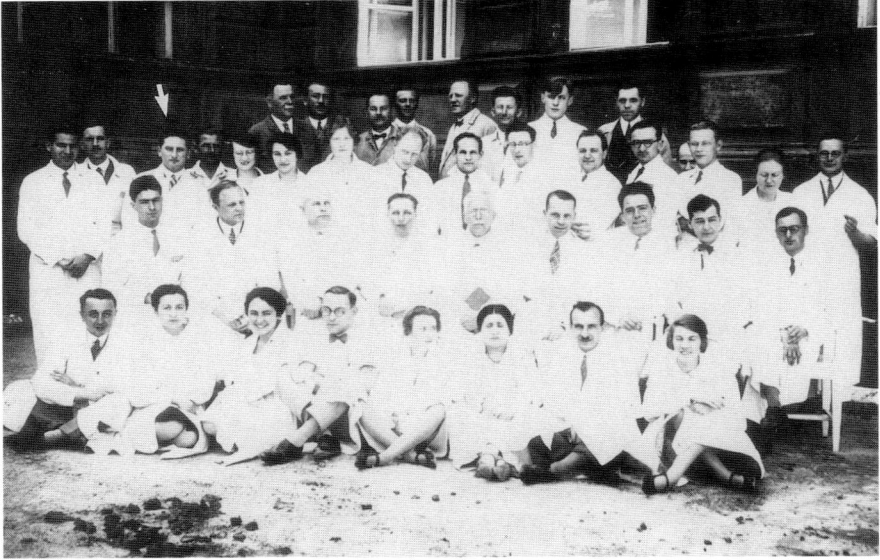

FIG. 9. Hans Popper (arrow) and his pathology colleagues in Vienna during the 1920s.
(Courtesy of Helmut Denk.)

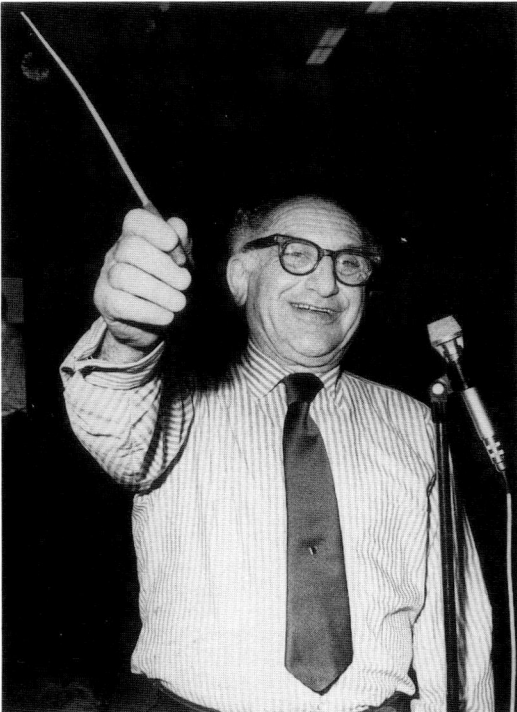

FIG. 10. Hans Popper conducting the brass orchestra one evening during the symposium on "Collagen Metabolism in the Liver," Freiburg i. Br., in 1973. Although submitted by Drs. Desmet, Bianchi, Falk, and others, this photograph was not one of Dr. Popper's favorite poses.

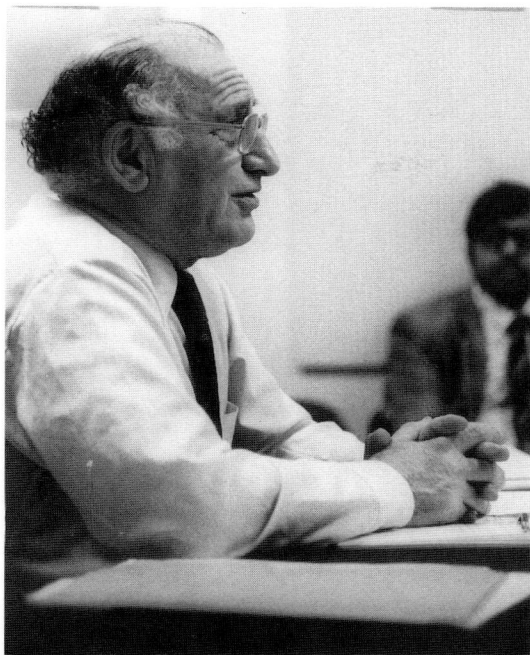

FIG. 11. Hans at meeting of the "gnomes," Leuven, 1976.
(Courtesy of V. J. Desmet.)

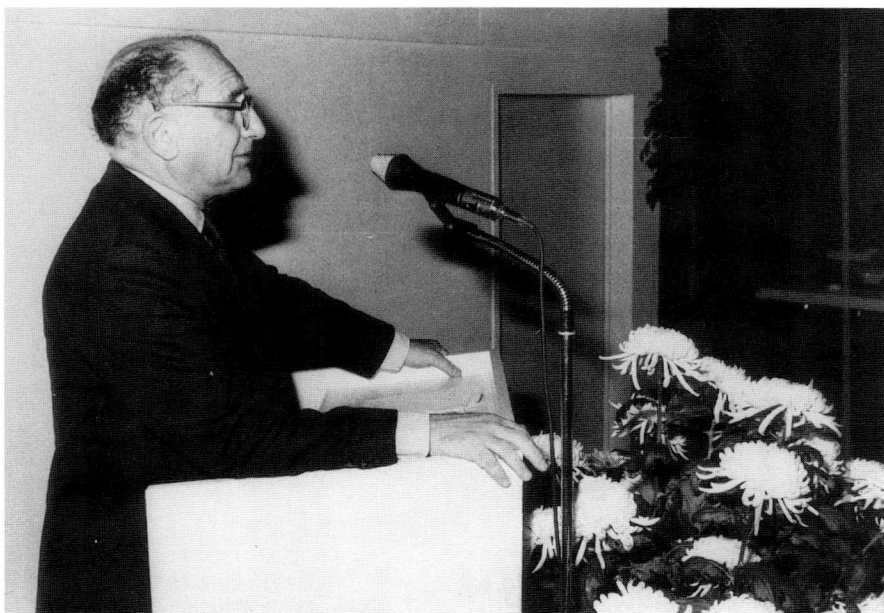

FIG. 12. Hans presiding over a Basel Liver Week.
(Courtesy of V. J. Desmet.)

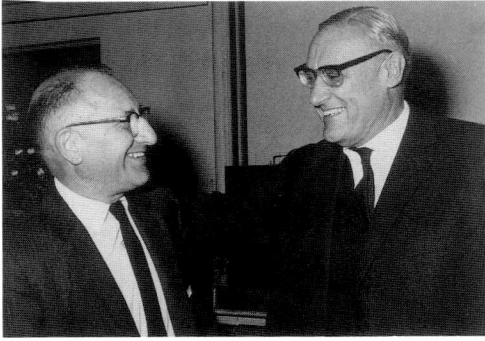

FIG. 13. Hans Popper with Ludwig Heilmeyer, Freiburg, October 1967.
(Courtesy of Herbert Falk.)

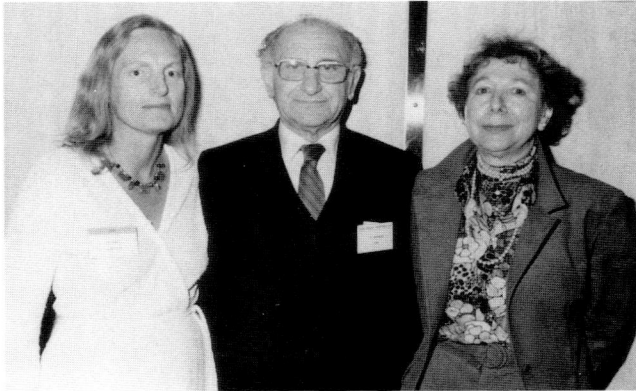

FIG. 14. Pauline Hall, Hans, and Lina Popper at the IASL/APASL meetings, Hong Kong, 1980. *(Courtesy of Pauline Hall.)*

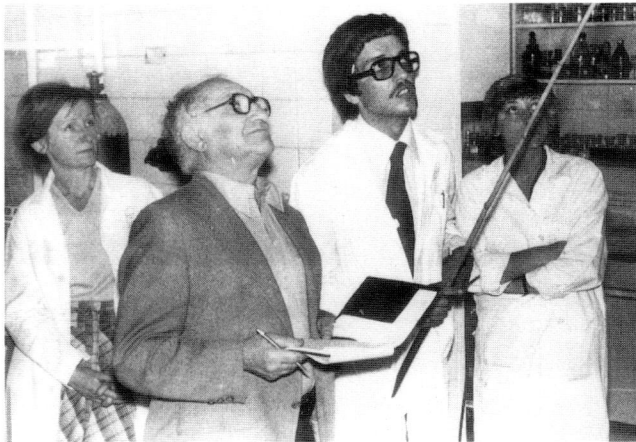

FIG. 15. Hans Popper reviews and discusses posters presented by staff doctors on the occasion of his visit to the First Institute of Pathology and Experimental Cancer Research, Semmelweis Medical University, Budapest, in 1980. *(Courtesy of Karoly Lapis.)*

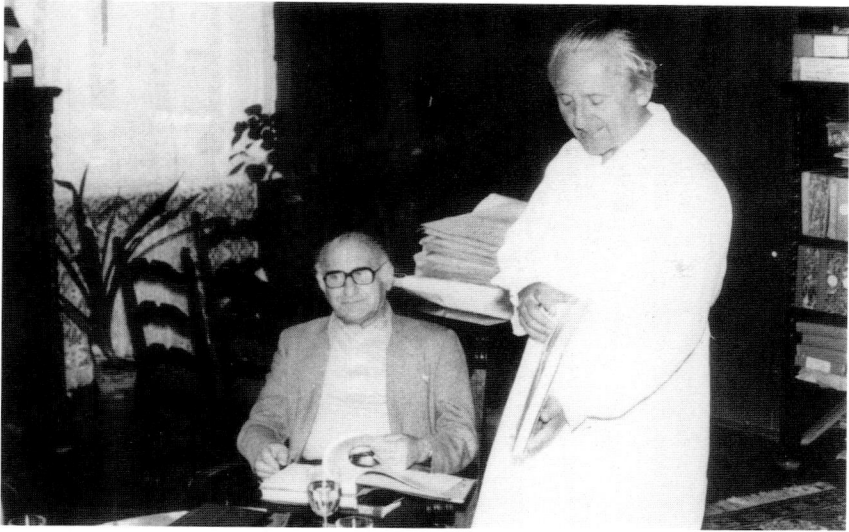

FIG. 16. Hans Popper and Dr. Lapis discussing the scientific activities of the First Institute of Pathology and Experimental Cancer Research, Semmelweis Medical University in Budapest in 1980.

(Courtesy of Karoly Lapis.)

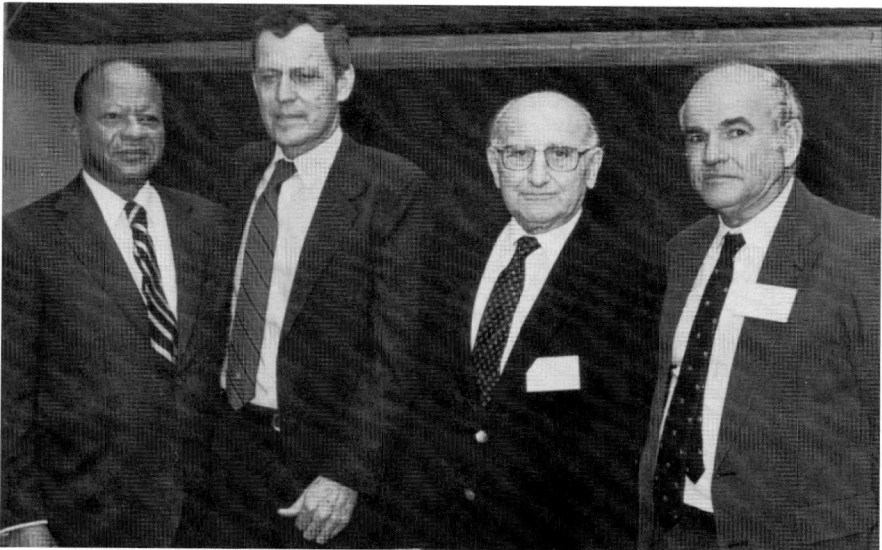

FIG. 17. Under the approving eye of Carroll M. Leevy (left), Hepatology Achievement Awards were presented at the first scientific symposium of the Sammy Davis, Jr., National Liver Institute to: Thomas Starzl, M.D., Ph.D., for developing a safe, effective method for liver transplantation in man; Hans Popper, M.D., Ph.D., for documenting the structural changes and pathobiology of hepatobiliary disease; and Baruch S. Blumberg, M.D., Ph.D., for basic contributions in identifying the hepatitis B virus and developing an effective vaccine.

(Courtesy of Carroll M. Leevy.)

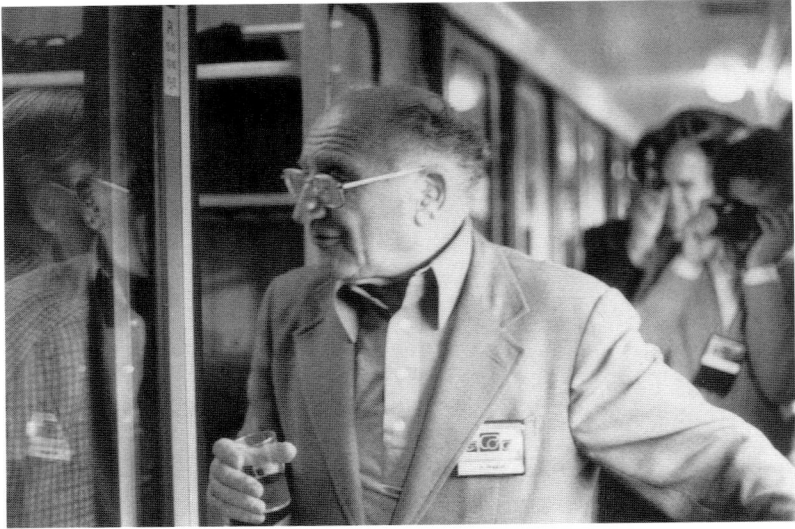

FIG. 18. Hans Popper on a train hurtling through the Swiss-German border, surrounded by hepatologic paparazzi. Basel Liver Week, 1978. *(Courtesy of Jay H. Lefkowitch.)*

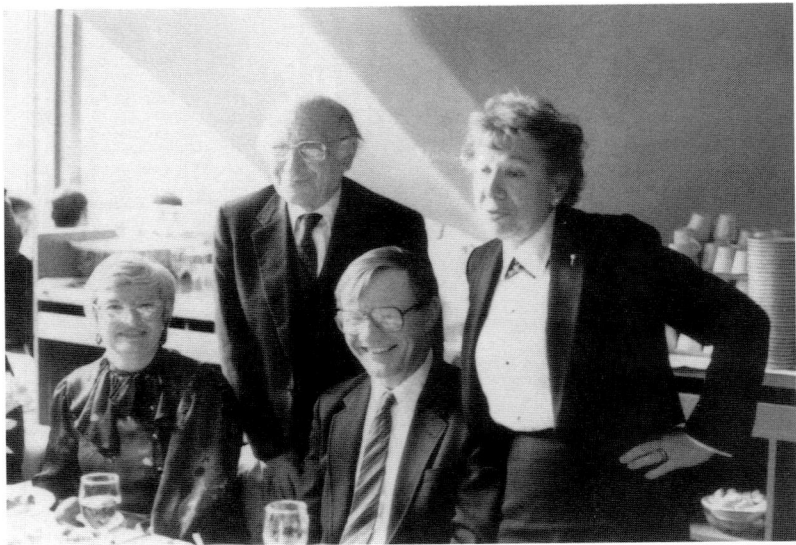

FIG. 19. Dinner at Avery Fisher Hall at Lincoln Center in New York City, May 12, 1983. Standing, Hans and Lina Popper. Seated, Mrs. Robert Glickman and Dr. Samuel French. *(Courtesy of Jay H. Lefkowitch.)*

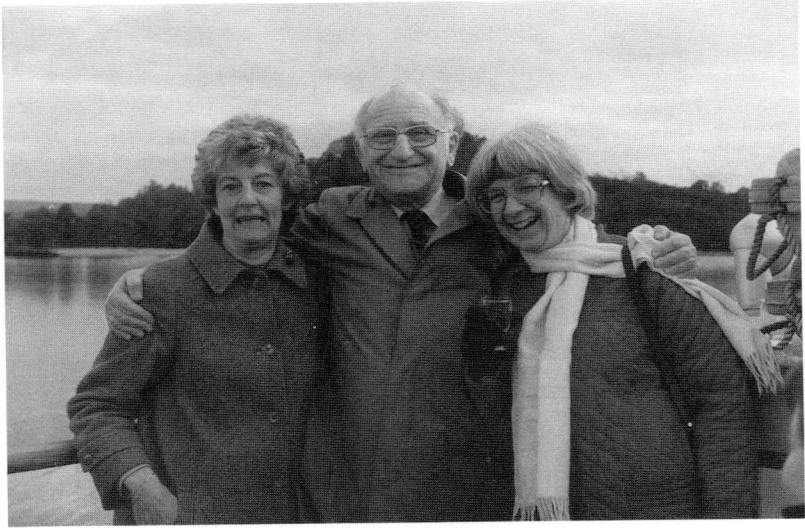

FIG. 20. Charming and charmed: Hans, Louise Scheuer (right), and Marjory MacSween (left), on Loch Lomond, 1982.
(Courtesy of Roddy MacSween.)

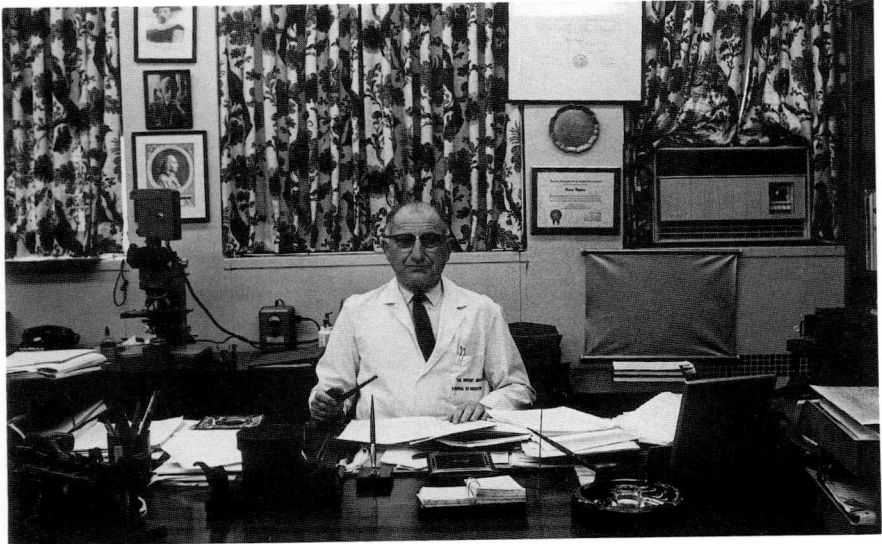

FIG. 21. Dr. Popper as Mount Sinai's pathologist-in-chief in his famous Atran office.
(Courtesy of Reba Nosoff.)

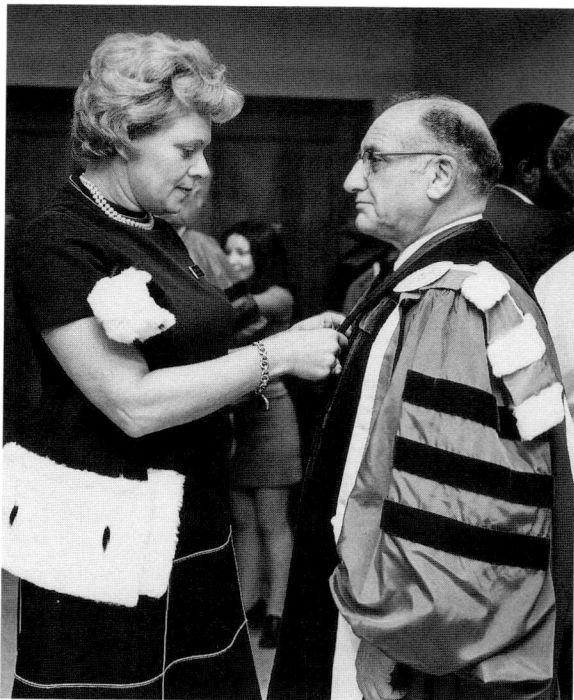

FIG. 22. Reba Nosoff helping Dr. Popper get ready for Commencement, Mount Sinai, 1972. *(Courtesy of Reba Nosoff.)*

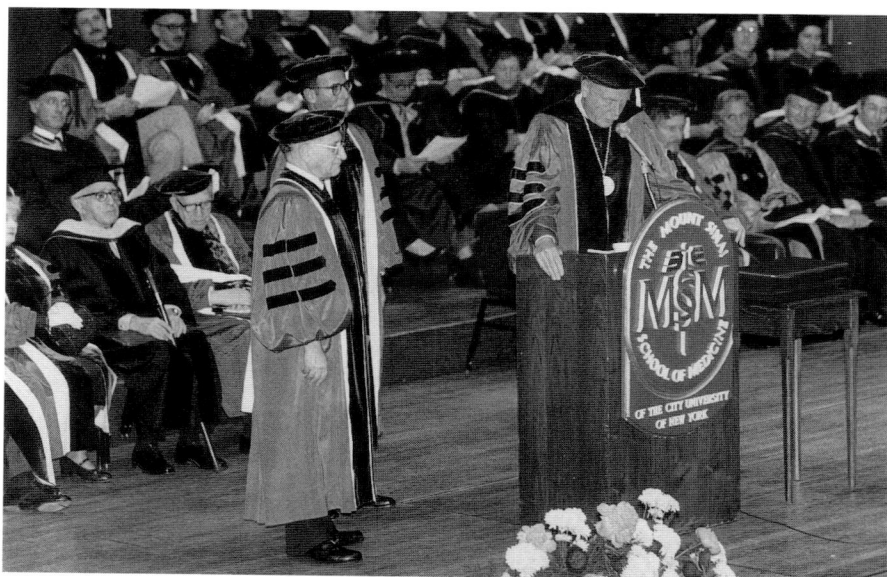

FIG. 23. Commencement at Mount Sinai, 1979. President Thomas Chalmers awards an honorary degree to Dr. Popper, his predecessor. *(Courtesy of Reba Nosoff.)*

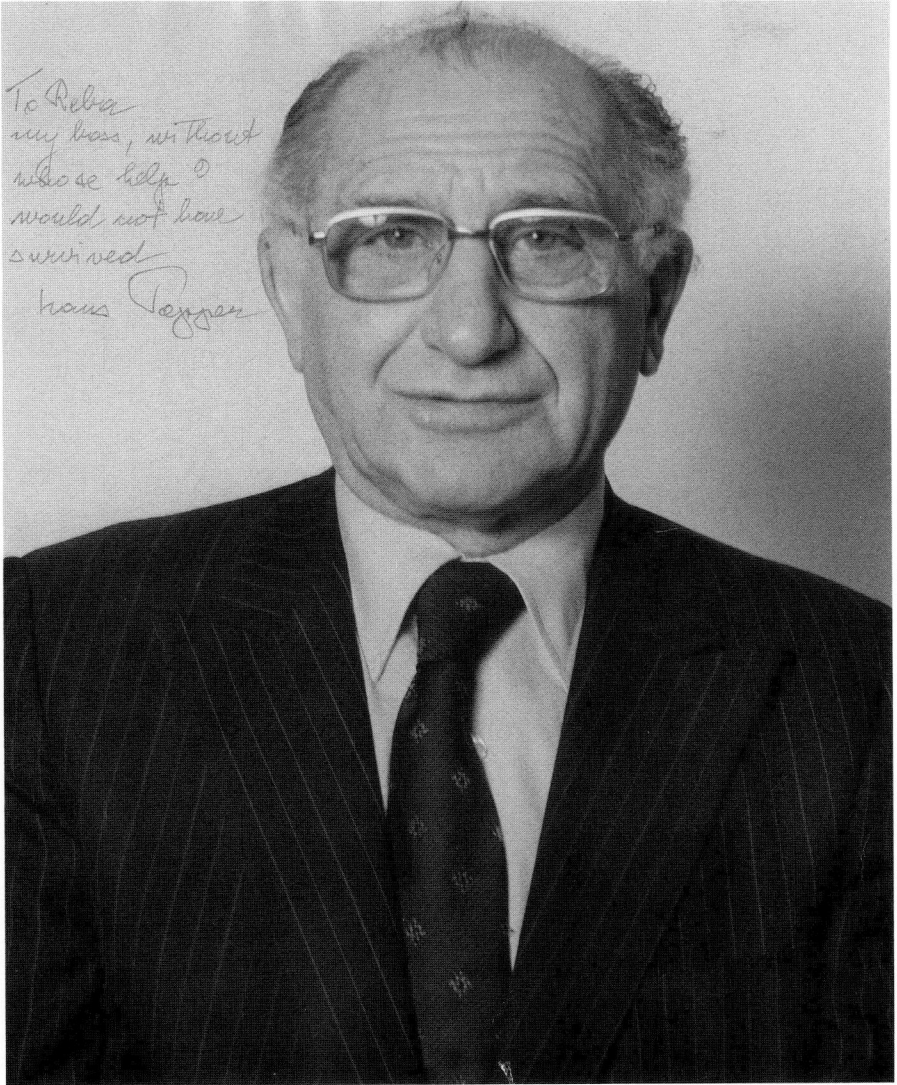

FIG. 24. Autographed photograph presented by Dr. Popper to Reba Nosoff.
(Courtesy of Reba Nosoff.)

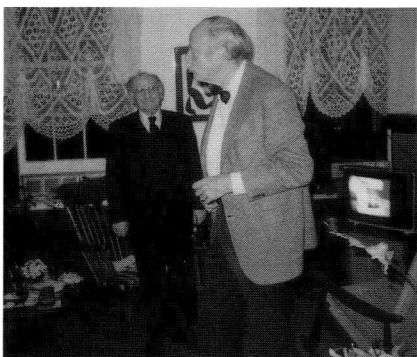

FIG. 25. Birthday dinner given by Reba Nosoff. Pictured: Dr. Popper and Dr. Chalmers.

(Courtesy of Reba Nosoff.)

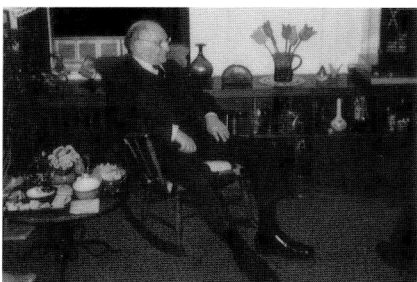

FIG. 26. Birthday dinner—Hans in his favorite chair—near the cream puffs.

(Courtesy of Reba Nosoff.)

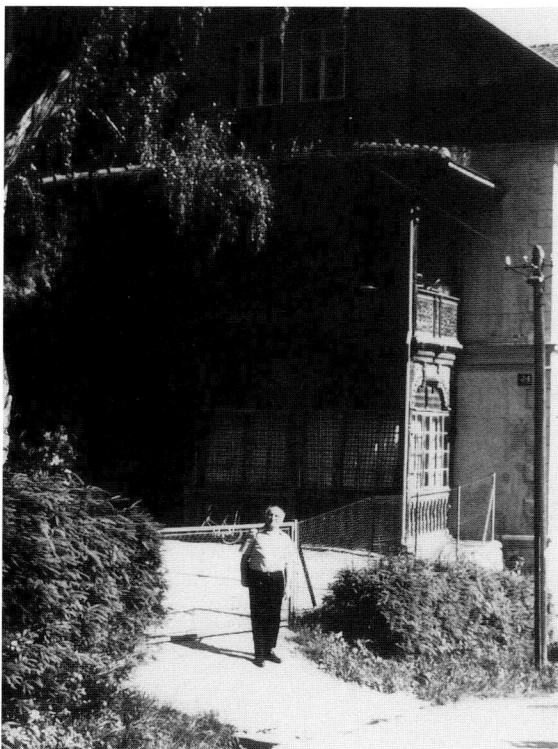

FIG. 27. Hans in front of the Popper pre-World War I summer vacation home at Reichenau, Austria, where early "word games" began. Photograph taken in the summer of 1976.

(Courtesy of Fenton Schaffner.)

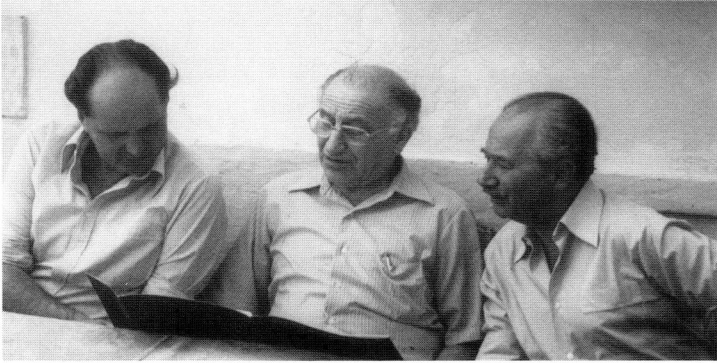

FIG. 28. Herbert Falk, Hans, and Heribert Thaler (left to right), all experts busy at "word games." *(Courtesy of Fenton Schaffner.)*

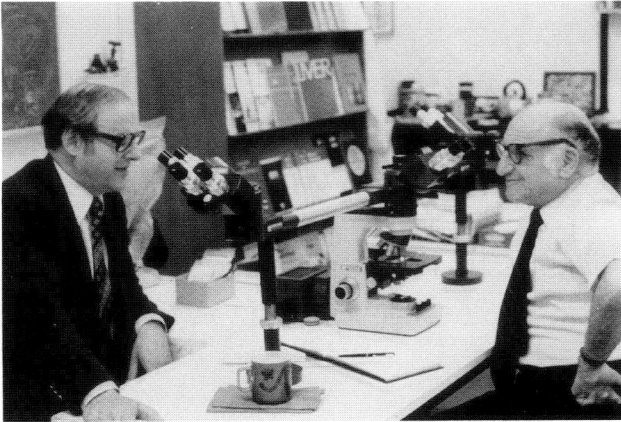

FIG. 29. Dr. Popper visits Dr. Scheuer in the latter's department, Royal Free Hospital, London, 1981. *(Courtesy of Peter J. Scheuer.)*

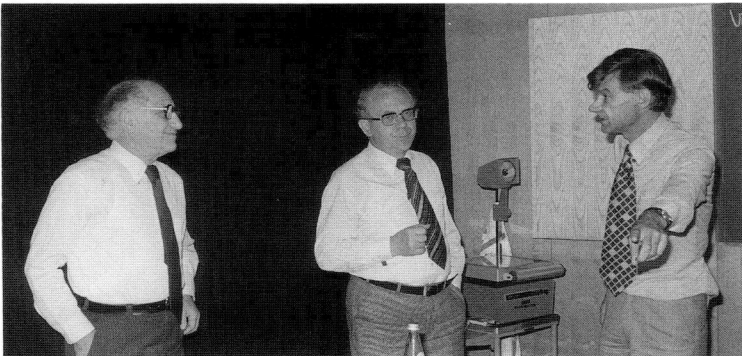

FIG. 30. The "gnomes of Zurich," 1978.
(Courtesy of Peter J. Scheuer.)

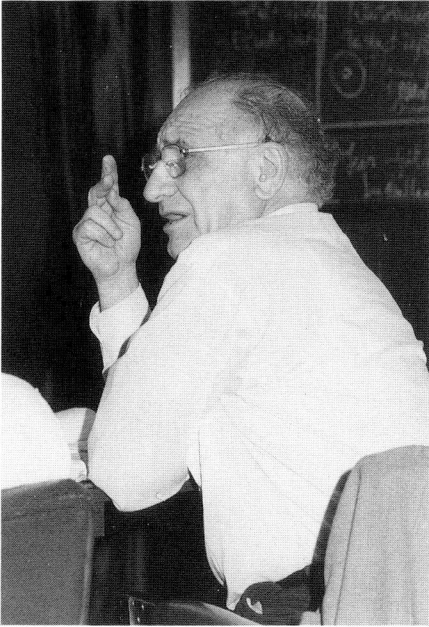

FIG. 31. Dr. Popper at a meeting of the "gnomes," London, 1979.
(Courtesy of Peter J. Scheuer.)

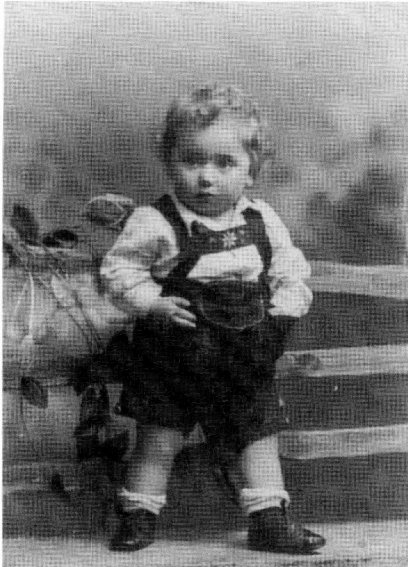

FIG. 32. Hans Popper at about age 2. It all began in Austria.
(Reprinted with permission from Hepatology 1989;9:670.)

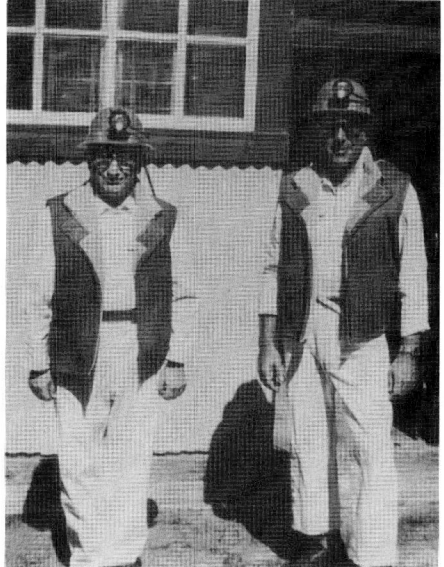

FIG. 33. Hans Popper and Fenton Schaffner. "Goldminers," 1972, Johannesburg, just prior to descending below 5,000 feet.
(Reprinted with permission from Hepatology 1989;9:672.)

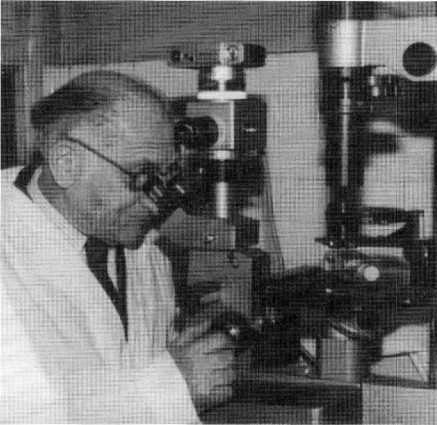

FIG. 34. Hans Popper, 1982. His
favorite pastime.
*(Reprinted with permission from
Hepatology 1989;9:670.)*

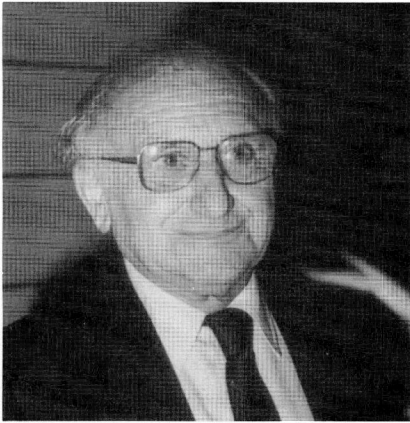

FIG. 35. Hans Popper, 1984, on the
occasion of receiving an honorary
degree at the University of Freiburg.
*(Reprinted with permission from
Hepatology 1989;9:669.)*

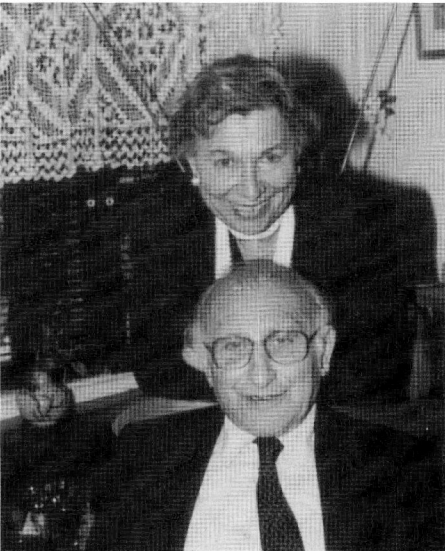

FIG. 36. Hans Popper at birthday party,
1984, with Lina Popper, his staunch
supporter and power behind the throne.
*(Reprinted with permission from
Hepatology 1989;9:674.)*

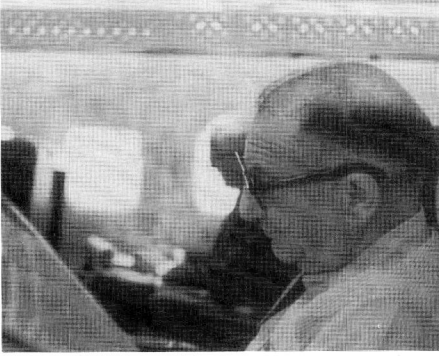

FIG. 37. Hans Popper, 1987. Airborne at 30,000 feet, his favorite reading room. *(Reprinted with permission from Hepatology 1989;9:671.)*

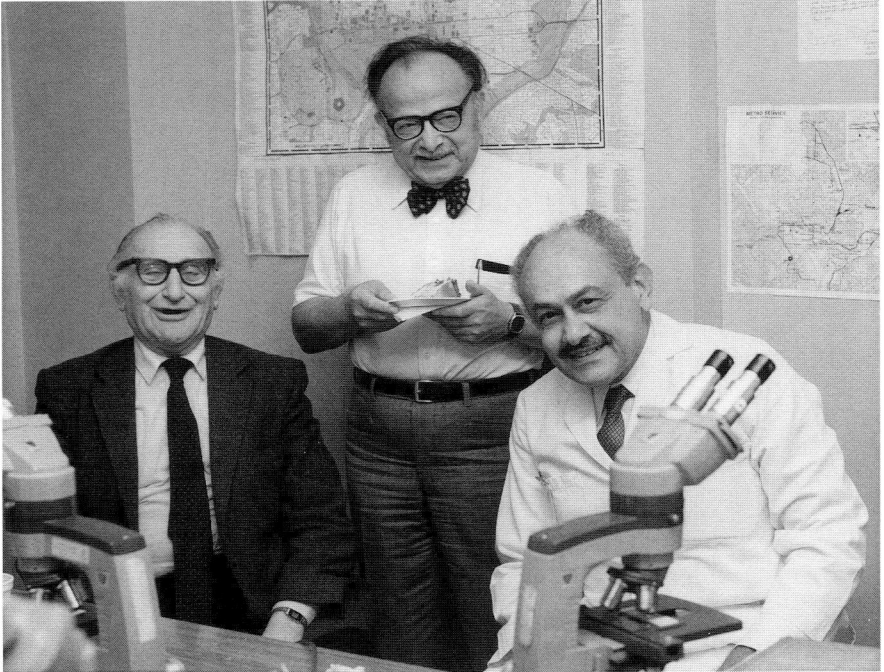

FIG. 38. Hans Popper, Hy Zimmerman, and Kamal Ishak celebrate Hans' 80th birthday at AFIP, 1983. *(Courtesy of Hyman Zimmerman and Kamal Ishak.)*

20

Karoly Lapis, Budapest

I first met Prof. Popper at a Falk Foundation Basel Liver Week. He made a deep impression on me not only with his excellent lectures but also with his brilliant summaries, in which he reviewed the main points of the presentations delivered during the meeting, emphasized the most important achievements, and outlined the problems to be solved next.

It especially impressed me that, despite his several engagements, he always visited the poster sections (see Fig. 15 in photo section) too, and he paid particular attention to the posters of the researchers coming from Eastern European countries. He always made useful, encouraging comments or constructive critical remarks to these authors. This was very important and stimulating for me and I presume for all my colleagues from the Eastern bloc.

Over the years, gradually a more and more close relationship developed between us, the result of which was that in 1980 he accepted our invitation and, together with his kind wife, Lina, he came to Budapest and visited our Institute. All the senior and junior members of the Institute looked forward to this visit with great enthusiasm and expectations; he lived up to all of them. In addition to delivering an excellent lecture, he provided us possibilities to have informal meetings too, during which we could discuss with him our problems and ask questions and solicit advice and encouragement concerning the new experiments we were about to launch. Visiting laboratory after laboratory, Prof. Popper became acquainted with the activity of our Institute and with the work, plans, and goals of the youngest researchers. He listened to their demonstrations with great interest. He was impressed that everyone in our Institute was fluent in English and that several colleagues spoke German as well. (See Fig. 16 in photo section.)

Those who knew him know that he was enthusiastically interested in liver pathology; it was this same enthusiastic interest he showed in everyday life, in culture and the cultural treasures of a country or city, and in the people of different nations. He knew a lot about the history and culture of Hungary, but he had a strong drive to learn even more. His increased interest in us had obviously originated from his knowledge of the history and culture of the Austro-Hungarian monarchy.

During their visit to Hungary Prof. Popper and his wife most enjoyed the beauty of the Danube Band and of Lake Balaton. I was especially glad that when we visited the city of Székesfehérvár, the ancient royal residence, we had the possibility of showing him the library of the Roman Catholic Church. He listened to the explanations of the bishop with great interest, and with even greater interest he leafed through the invaluable books that represented rarities of Hungarian culture and church history.

I dare say that during his visit a sincerely friendly relationship developed with the seniors and an almost fatherly one with the young colleagues, which resulted in some of us having the pleasure and honor of visiting him in his laboratory at Mount Sinai. On the walls of his laboratory and his study we could admire pictures that delineated every important moment or achievement of the history of medicine in the 20th century.

In 1984–1985, when I worked more than a year at the National Cancer Institute as a Fogarty Scholar-in-Residence, I regularly attended the liver seminars given by Prof. Popper every month, where I sometimes was fortunate enough to witness "in status nascendi" how a theory was taking shape and was developing in his mind. One of these seminars ended rather late, and I had the privilege of taking him to the airport. We had some hours until the departure of the plane; thus, he invited my wife and me to the Cosmos Club in Washington for dinner. The walls of the club were decorated with pictures of prominent American scholars. While we were having our aperitifs, Prof. Popper gave us concise and witty descriptions of the contributions that these people had made to the development of the different fields of science and technology. This remains an unforgettable evening for both my wife and me.

It was my greatest regret that, although I received a personal invitation, I could not go to Vienna to the celebration of his 80th birthday. Luckily, after this I still met and had discussions with him several times.

I am quite convinced that every member of our Institute as well as all the Hungarian hepatologists will pay homage to his memory and remember him with sincere affection.

21

Carroll M. Leevy, Newark

HANS POPPER AND SAMMY DAVIS, JR.

In 1987, a committee of distinguished scientists and laymen selected Hans Popper as a recipient of the Sammy Davis, Jr., Hepatology Achievement Award (see Fig. 17 in photo section). Dr. Popper was singled out for his lifelong contributions to an understanding of the pathophysiology of liver disease and his unique dedication to improving prevention, recognition, and management of liver disease. Sammy Davis, Jr., was especially interested in the social aspects of liver disease and was particularly intrigued by Hans' focus on this area of medicine (1). In organizing the Sammy Davis, Jr., National Liver Institute, which has increased public awareness of diseases of the liver, Sammy wanted to help realize Dr. Popper's goal—to educate the population on prevention of liver disease and, at the same time, improve ability to detect and treat it. This commentary describes some of the interactions of Hans Popper with liver disease through what has become the National Liver Institute memorializing Sammy Davis, Jr.

DIGESTIVE DISEASE EDUCATION   Hans Popper and his medical associates and Sammy Davis, Jr., and his colleagues all attempted to organize a strong lay support group for liver and other digestive diseases. Dr. Popper was founder and continuous leader of the American and International Associations for Study of the Liver. He was also central in the effort that led to the organization of the Digestive Diseases Foundation with chapters in each of the 50 states in the early 1970s. Unfortunately, lack of agreement between various organizations prevented full realization of this goal. Hans' work

87

with the Steering (Scope) Committee, established while I was president of the American Association for Study of the Liver, gave hepatology the boost it needed—special attention to lay and professional education; organization of the American Liver Foundation; initiation of an annual Refresher Course on Advances in Liver Disease; and the establishment of a monthly journal. Working with other digestive disease organizations, this group helped arrange for Congress to establish a Commission on Digestive Diseases, which charted the course for this discipline in the United States, and tried to create an Institute for Digestive Diseases, still needed at the National Institutes of Health.

BIOMEDICAL RESEARCH   I first met Dr. Popper at the 1957 meeting of the American Association for Study of the Liver (2). Following my report on investigations of the hepatic circulation, he invited me to visit him; this began a series of fruitful conversations and conjoint efforts on research in liver disease. These meetings, which extended over the next 30 years, were often in the company of his devoted wife Lina and my family in various parts of the world. Thus, many of the basic concepts of the pathogenesis, sequence, and treatment of portal hypertension, measurement of hepatic and portal blood flow, and the use of clearance techniques to detect liver disease emerged from such dialogue with Hans in which Charles Mendenhall, Gustav Paumgartner, and Robert Stone were participants. In organizational activities, Hans and I shared in the problems attendant to establishing a new medical school. My effort, which was stimulated by a desire to improve education, patient care, and research for patients with liver disease, began in 1952 and faced much difficulty in establishing a Catholic Medical School at the Jersey City Medical Center. After 1960, I consulted Hans frequently on matters including conversion of the medical school to a state institution, transfer of the school from Jersey City to Newark, which helped precipitate the 1967 riots; and, finally, merging all of medical education in New Jersey under one umbrella as a Health Science University (3). Dr. Popper was always optimistic, believing New Jersey would survive its multiple problems and long dependence on others for medical education and health care. He was a prime advisor in getting me to turn down attractive offers to go elsewhere and accept the chairmanship of the Department of Medicine at the New Jersey Medical School. For his numerous accomplishments, including advice and assistance in the development of the medical school, which included many visits to both Jersey City and Newark, Dr. Popper received an Honorary Doctor of Science Degree from the University of Medicine and Dentistry of New Jersey.

After a period at the Thorndike with Drs. Charlie Davidson, Rudi Schmid, and Richard McDonald, my attention turned to studies of hepatic

DNA and collagen synthesis. Returning to New Jersey, Dr. Popper again became an advisor on these studies, which defined the kinetics of cell replication in hepatitis, cirrhosis, and liver disease. Using protozoologic methods, developed by Drs. Herman Baker and Oscar Frank at the New Jersey Medical School, it was found that a deficiency of folic acid, vitamin B_6, vitamin B_{12}, and zinc reduced hepatic DNA synthesis (4). With Hans' help, we used this finding to get the FDA to add folic acid to commercially available vitamin preparations to prevent both the macrocytic anemia and aregenerative phases of liver injury characteristic of malnourished alcoholics. Subsequently, it was found that protein and androgenic anabolic steroids increased hepatic DNA synthesis and liver regeneration and a fibrogenic factor which contributes to collagen deposition in chronic liver disease was discovered. Development of an *in vitro* perfusion technique to evaluate hepatic DNA and collagen synthesis in percutaneous liver biopsies led to many unexpected discoveries that allowed us to systematically evaluate the various therapeutic modalities advocated to stimulate liver repair. Dr. Popper encouraged us to pursue our studies, which demonstrated a humoral factor in liver injury; however, we were not able to obtain that "magic potion" that might be a partial answer to interrupting progressive liver failure.

During a trip to London and Stockholm with Hans, we explored the concept of immunologic reactivity in noninfectious diseases. In consultation with Dr. Popper, the New Jersey group initially consisting of Drs. Hsu, Sorrell, Zetterman, Maximoto, Kanagasundaram, and Kakumu explored the possibility that immunologic reactivity was responsible for alcoholic hepatitis. This new genre of research presented to Hans Popper by Dr. Michael Sorrell led him to say this was most exciting and revolutionary. It was agreed that an immunologic abnormality existed from both *in vivo* and *in vitro* studies; however, the specific mechanism and implications have remained unsettled. Autologous liver from patients with alcoholic hepatitis added to lymphocytes caused release of cytotoxic, fibrogenic, migration inhibition factor, and other lymphokines. Isolated, purified Mallory bodies were assumed to be antigenic; this thesis was supported by development of Mallory body-specific monoclonal antibody, which blocks leukocyte migration (5). In my last conversation with Hans, he said he believed Mallory bodies were antigenic and urged the New Jersey group to pursue this hypothesis and develop a serologic test to readily recognize persons who harbor Mallory bodies.

DIAGNOSTIC CRITERIA FOR HEPATOLOGY In 1972, as president of the International Association for Study of the Liver, the World Health Organization asked me to help standardize nomenclature of diseases of the liver and biliary tract. Dr. Popper, Dr. Sherlock, and I met, but it was apparent that this required long, continuous effort. We had two unique objectives: obtaining agreement among the international community of experts in hepatology, and getting students, housestaff, and practitioners to talk the same language (6). Shortly afterwards, using the same mechanism, the FDA standardized detection of hepatotoxicity due to chemicals and drugs, the legal device for regulating production of drugs that have predictable or unpredictable toxicity in America (7). These efforts were widely distributed in other languages; however, no revisions occurred until Sammy Davis, Jr., became interested in helping achieve the original objective of the World Health Organization. Looking at English editions of these books, he said, "We must update them." Following the lead of Hans Popper, this interest led to the organization of the Sammy Davis, Jr., National Liver Institute with a major focus on educating both laity and professionals. The newest edition of diagnostic criteria, which now also addresses the complex issue of prognosis—with attention to the influence of medical and surgical therapy on quality of life and longevity—would please both Hans and Sammy.

The physician, Hans Popper, and the entertainer, Sammy Davis, Jr., dreamed the same dream; both sought excellence and compassion. Both believed it necessary for society to establish models and encourage all peoples to work together, eliminating all vestiges of racism and politicism. Both Hans and Sammy were deeply affected by impoverished and undereducated people suffering from liver disease. Hans, as Sammy, was an optimist, a leader whose life on earth will forever change mortal existence, helping address an often neglected disease that involves much of mankind. Hans was fully engulfed in the discovery of new knowledge through science to help eliminate the scourge of disease. Sammy attempted to make life a delightful, hopeful episode free of suffering from which good dreams are made. Together they achieved much for their generation and generations to come. In the planned homebase for the Sammy Davis, Jr., National Liver Institute, an area will be devoted to a history of the development and developers of hepatology. Hans Popper has already been assigned a special place in this module.

References

1. Popper H, Davidson CD, Leevy CM, Schaffner F. The social impact of liver disease. *N Engl J Med* 1969; 281:1455.
2. Leevy CM. Organization of research in new medical schools. In: Proceedings of the International Symposium on the Role of Research in Medical Education, Fogarty International Center. Washington, DC: U.S. Government Printing Office, 1971:No. 7, p. 147.
3. Leevy CM, Gliedman ML. Practical and research value of hepatic vein catheterization. *N Engl J Med* 1958; 258:696–738.

4. Leevy CM. *In vitro* studies of hepatic DNA synthesis in percutaneous liver biopsy specimens from man. *J Lab Clin Med* 1963; 61:761.
5. Leevy CB, Sameshima Y, Yoshioka K, Leevy CM, Kanagasundaram N, Unoura M. Use of specific monoclonal antibody to detect Mallory bodies in liver disease. *JAAMP* 1990; 1:24.
6. Leevy CM, Popper H, Sherlock S. Diseases of the liver and biliary tract, standardization of nomenclature, diagnostic criteria and diagnostic methodology, Fogarty International Center. Washington, DC: U.S. Government Printing Office, 1977: No. 22.
7. Davidson CS, Leevy CM, Chamberlayne EC. Guidelines for detection of drug and chemical induced hepatotoxicity, Fogarty International Center. Washington, DC: U.S. Government Printing Office, 1979: No. 79.

22

Jay H. Lefkowitch, New York

The unvarnished truth is that, as a medical student, I never understood a word of Dr. Popper's lectures on the liver. Nor did any of my classmates. It was some strange Viennese-American *urtext* on the liver—cryptic, indecipherable, and unfathomable. Mind you, we all had expected more. After all, this was the great liver pathologist from Mount Sinai who had been imported uptown to lecture at Columbia. With this inauspicious beginning, it is truly a wonder that I ever became interested in the liver. As it turned out, I later learned not only to speak and comprehend his unique dialect but also to relish every opportunity of sharing his counsel.

Hans stayed young to the end. He found continual inspiration in new scientific information. Being with young people provided him his personal fountain of youth.

One of my early remembrances of Hans was from 1978, on a train speeding through the Swiss–German border. It was one of Dr. Falk's Basel Liver Week outings in which thousands of hepatologists from all over the globe would be transported (on our version of the Orient Express) to an enormous and festive beer hall, complete with lederhosen, for a banquet dinner. It was like being on that train with Michael Redgrave and Dame May Whitty in *The Lady Vanishes*, only the players were different. Hans carried his international persona with him even on that train trip. I was passing from one car into the next on the train and nearly walked into Dr. Popper directly in front of me (see Fig. 18 in photo section), surrounded by hepatologic paparazzi.

Near Hans was a rather formidable looking woman with auburn-red hair (not shown in the photograph) who would momentarily be engaged in an intense discussion with him. They each had a drink in hand, and, as the train sped around a bend, their dialogue about the liver began. It was my first encounter with Dame Sheila Sherlock and Hans Popper talking shop.

It was Hans who recommended me to study with Prof. Peter J. Scheuer at the Royal Free Hospital in London. Peter had himself studied with Hans, so there was a great sense of continuity in my liver training. As a mentor, Peter was (and is) nonpareil, and I am ever grateful to Hans for pointing me in the direction of London.

In my first decade of liver work after 1978, it was an ever-increasing source of comfort to know that Hans was here in New York for consultation. He relished talking about so many things—diagnostic problems, the latest cell biology he had read about in *Science* or *Nature*, political (i.e., medical school) dirt—all with animation, albeit sprinkled with references to his arthritic pains, angina, and overcommitments to give lectures out of town. Don't we all recall sitting in anticipation outside his office chatting with Clare and Lore, while waiting for our audience with Hans? No matter how busy, though, his eyes lit up at the prospect of a challenging biopsy.

Hans' powers with the H&E slide were, most of the time, uncanny. Of course, he never wanted a word of history about the patient when consulted on a difficult biopsy. About a year or so before he died, I regretted not bringing a young resident or a student with me to witness Hans in action. The case in question was a young alcoholic man with AIDS who had some peculiar vascular ectatic lesions in the portal tracts, which I suspected were probably Kaposi's sarcoma. I walked into Hans office, sat down, and handed him the slide. As usual, he turned around in his ample brown chair to look at the slide on the microscope. A minute elapsed. Then, as his chair turned around, Hans leaned back, arms akimbo, grinning broadly as he said to me matter-of-factly, "So, zis is an alcoholic with AIDS?" The "simple H&E man," as he called himself, had done it again.

I have so many wonderful memories of Hans, and of Lina and Hans. In 1985, I held an exhibit of some of my paintings at the National Arts Club and enjoyed having friends and colleagues come to see it. Lina and Hans were in Munich that week at a liver meeting and I didn't expect to see them there. However, the last day of my show, having just come off a plane from Europe with jet lag, they both came downtown to see the exhibit before it was dismantled. You don't forget things like that.

Hans joined us at Columbia P & S for many postgraduate courses in liver pathology during the 1980s, and, on the occasion of his 80th birthday in 1983, we inaugurated a Hans Popper Lectureship in Liver Pathology. That year, the faculty celebrated with a concert and dinner in Avery Fisher Hall at Lincoln Center. Once again, it was a family affair, a time to share in science and friendship. I like the photograph I took that night at the restaurant in Avery Fisher Hall (Fig. 19). It shows Hans as I think we would all like to remember him: looking wise, with Lina at his side, enjoying culture, and vigorously engaged with colleagues in the pursuit of new hepatologic understanding.

23

Charles S. Lieber, New York

My first exposure to Hans Popper was in 1958 at the annual meeting of the American Association for the Study of Liver Diseases in Chicago: what was most impressive about Hans Popper was the extraordinary breadth of his expertise, ranging from the ultrastructure of the liver to an unchallenged mastership of light microscopy and a keen grasp of the most intricate concepts of biochemistry and molecular biology. To a budding hepatologist, he was the role model par excellence.

Between 1958 and 1968, my contacts with Hans Popper were limited to those of scientific meetings, but in 1968 this all changed with the advent of The Mount Sinai School of Medicine, the founding of which was largely due to the great vision and tremendous energy of this one man. He profusely used his intellectual charms to enlist a score of new faculty members, and he was most influential in attracting me to this new school. But his commitment did not stop with successful recruitment. For the subsequent two decades, he actively participated in our teaching program. His clinical–pathological liver conferences soon became legendary: once a month, he spent 1 hour with us reviewing blindly our most challenging liver biopsy cases. His capacity to derive an accurate clinical history from the morphologic changes was uncanny. Not infrequently, he derived more clinical information from a slide than had been gathered in hours of bedside interviews. Never have I seen anyone come even close to his extraordinary diagnostic skills. These monthly meetings were also the occasion for vivid and enlightening updating on ongoing hepatology research worldwide, providing us with a one-man journal club. He was not only a source of key information but also gave us priceless critical evaluation. We are now sorely missing Hans Popper's

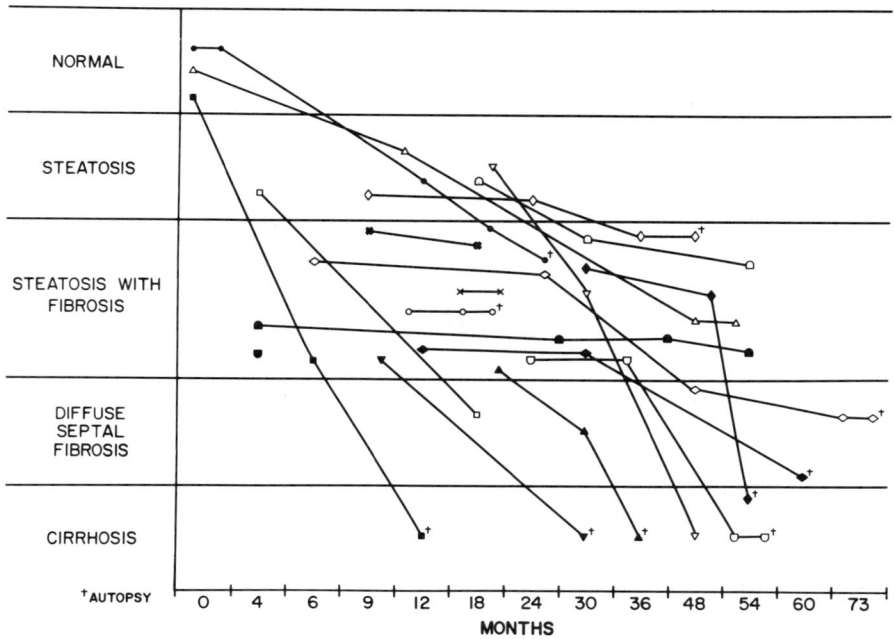

Sequential development of alcoholic liver injury. The most severe lesion is recorded individually for each time period in 18 baboons fed alcohol up to 6 years. (Reprinted with permission from Popper H, Lieber CS. Histogenesis of alcoholic fibrosis and cirrhosis in the baboon. *Am J Pathol* 1980;98:695–716.)

extraordinary insights, which allowed him to easily glean from a tremendous wealth of information those few points that turned out subsequently to have been trendsetting. His knowledge and insight easily matched the expertise of many multidisciplinary centers and their teams of experts.

The scientific discussions Hans Popper generated in his monthly sessions with us created a very stimulating atmosphere, which eventually evolved into a rewarding scientific collaboration. We had reported before that, even in the absence of dietary deficiencies, alcohol can produce fatty livers and ultrastructural changes in man and experimental animals and the ultimate stage of alcoholic cirrhosis in the baboon. However, the dogma that alcohol is not a hepatotoxin and that its effects on the liver were due merely to malnutrition was so strongly entrenched that the nature of our findings in the baboon were seriously questioned. Our biochemical expertise was not challenged, but our morphologic skills were not universally accepted. To lay to rest any possible doubts, input from an unimpeachable and universally respected pathologist was needed. Hans Popper generously consented to study blindly all of our tissues, starting *de novo* with the blocks and proceeding with his own stainings. This study not only firmly established that, even when associated with an adequate diet, ethanol can produce cirrhosis but also, as we had anticipated, Hans took the opportunity to develop a most comprehensive analysis of the pathologic development of the fibrotic lesion. Through a detailed study of all the intermediate stages, he succeeded in reconstructing the change of normal liver to cirrhosis by putting together all of his observations obtained in our entire baboon colony (see graph on the opposite page). Through his meticulous study of a large number of samples and sequential analysis of the tissue changes, Dr. Popper was able to define the progression of alcoholic liver injury from fatty liver to cirrhosis and to infer the histogenesis of fibrosis. His reconstruction of the developing lesion clearly established that fibrosis and cirrhosis can evolve even in the absence of alcoholic hepatitis, as defined by necrosis and inflammation (characterized by polymorphonuclear infiltration). This collaborative study also vividly illustrated Hans Popper's extraordinary flexibility, the hallmark of a true scientist. In spite of his occasional "Herr Professor" demeanor, he had the great capacity to abandon established ideas and to embrace new concepts, even some he himself had originally rejected. Prior to this endeavor with the baboon, Dr. Popper had espoused the prevailing dogma that alcoholic hepatitis was a necessary precursor stage of cirrhosis and a *sine qua non* of the development of that complication in alcoholic liver disease. When his own observations in the baboon showed a clear progression to cirrhosis in the absence of *bona fide* alcoholic hepatitis, he did not hesitate to reject the views he himself had many times expressed and published on the topic and became a strong advocate of the concept that, in addition to and independently of alcoholic hepatitis, other pathways may lead to alcoholic cirrhosis. The rich description of the perivenular lesion in that model and the reconstructed sequential analysis of the fibrotic change (see graph) provided us with a strong impetus to pursue, in man, our search for precirrhotic lesions other than alcoholic hepatitis. The perivenular fibrosis that was shown in the baboon to be indicative of the start of the fibrotic process was then found later in man to have predictive value in those individuals who are particularly prone to rapidly develop cirrhosis on continuation of drinking. Dr. Popper also described in detail the striking ballooning and other alterations of the hepatocyte produced by alcohol. This in turn was consistent with the importance of protein retention and swelling of the hepatocyte and associated alterations of the cytoskeleton, which we had previously reported in the rat and incriminated as possible factors leading to necrosis. These findings also led us to focus more intensely on mechanisms whereby collagen synthesis and fibrosis might be stimulated in a more direct fashion. Thus, it became clear that fibrosis and cirrhosis are not merely passive responses to inflammation and necrosis, but might result, at least in part, from direct effects of alcohol and its metabolites on collagen production and fibrogenesis. Indeed, we subsequently showed that acetaldehyde, the metabolite of ethanol, does in fact stimulate collagen production in myofibroblasts isolated from the baboon liver. The respective roles of the various cells of the liver in collagen formation is, now, of course the subject of a widely explored and productive area of scientific investigation.

One other major specific stimulus that Hans Popper provided was the realization of the importance of the fat-storing cells (also called Ito cells or lipocytes) in the pathogenesis of fibrosis. These vitamin A storing cells had been close to Dr. Popper's heart since the pioneering work he had completed four decades before, in the early 1940s, on the relationship between serum and liver vitamin A, the visualization of vitamin A in rat organs by fluorescence microscopy, and changes of vitamin A distribution in choline deficiency. These early insights in possible relationships between vitamin A and liver pathology were the forerunners of our more recent studies that eventually led to the discovery of the extraordinarily low vitamin A levels in alcoholic liver injury, even at its earliest stages. This in turn prompted us to elucidate the role of enhanced vitamin A breakdown under these conditions, which was found to be due, at least in part, to the induction of two hitherto unrecognized pathways of retinol catabolism in liver microsomes. It is Dr. Popper's visionary insight in the pathophysiologic meaning of morphologic changes that prompted him to recognize the potential importance of the lipocytes in the fibrotic process and that provided an invaluable stimulus that led us, as well as a score of other investigators, to attempt to delineate the role these cells play in the production of collagen and the genesis of cirrhosis.

These glimpses of some specific major scientific areas where Dr. Popper had a decisive impact on the orientation of our own research do not give full justice to his enriching influence. Through his "Rapid Abstracts," the entire field benefited from his unique capacity to sort the grain from the shaft. His volumes, *Progress in Liver Diseases*, provided continuing education for the hepatologist. The symposia he organized represented turning points and starting levels for the most exciting developments in the field of hepatology for almost half a century. But momentous as these accomplishments may be, they are dwarfed by the wealth of information and stimulation with which Hans Popper enriched my life for more than four decades and the warmth of his friendship for the last 20 years. He will be sorely missed and never forgotten.

24

Ian R. Mackay, Clayton

HEPATIC AUTOIMMUNITY, CHRONIC HEPATITIS, HEPATOCELLULAR
CANCER, AND THE AGING LIVER

Can reminiscences of the scientific contributions of the legendary Hans Popper be accommodated by a single volume of tribute? An encyclopedia of hepatology would be more appropriate!

My personal encounters with Hans Popper touched on mere segments of his vast experience in the physiology and pathology of the liver. These began when, as a naive research fellow at the University of Washington, Seattle, in 1952, I was sent on a "grand tour" of North American centers of excellence in hepatology, during the course of which I was to meet several great figures: Hans Popper was foremost among these. He was then pathologist at the Cook County Hospital, Chicago, and his welcome to me typified his ethos: hospitable and boundless enthusiasm for dialogue with any visitor prepared to reciprocate Hans' passion for hepatic histopathology.

After my return to Melbourne in 1955, I was working in an institute directed to basic immunology and in a unit with a particular interest in liver disease, including chronic hepatitis. Thus, the "stars were right" for an initiative in the immunology of hepatitis, a new field at that time. This led to my description of lupoid (autoimmune) hepatitis, to identify an unusual type of chronic hepatitis that was being recognized in several centers in the 1950s. The idea of autoimmunity as a cause of chronic hepatitis aroused much skepticism at that time, but it was heartening that Hans Popper, who liked new ideas, became quite sympathetic to the concept. This may have been because of his preceding interest in the chemical pathology of cirrhosis, and particularly in abnormalities that reflected changes in serum globulins. Indeed, Hans Popper, the immunochemist, was the first to document clearly that persistent gamma-globulin elevation was indicative of transition of hepatitis to cirrhosis even in the presence of normal hepatic function tests (*J Lab Clin Med* 1950; 35:391 and *Gastroenterology* 1951; 17:138).

Accordingly, Hans Popper and colleagues quickly turned their attention to immunohistochemistry, an infant science in the early 1960s, and demonstrated local formation of gamma globulin by immunofluorescence in the liver in chronic hepatitis and postnecrotic cirrhosis, reported in 1960. This local formation of gamma was postulated to be "in reticuloendothelial cells showing transition to plasma cells" (B lymphocytes were not known then) and the possibility was considered "that the gamma globulin formed may represent antibody to liver cell breakdown products" (*J Exp Med* 1960; 111:285). This tacit acceptance of autodestruction as a cause of liver cell death led to Dr. Popper's designation of the morphologic expression of this. So emerged the description of piecemeal necrosis. "The type of necrosis in chronic liver disease which correlates well qualitatively and roughly quantitatively with the presence of γ-globulin containing cells [in the liver] is 'piecemeal necrosis,' characterized by necrosis or disappearance of liver cells predominantly on the lobular or nodular periphery, and associated with the accumulation of lymphocytes, plasma cells and histocytes" (*Lab Invest* 1962; 11:150). Hans Popper subsequently deprecated the overuse of the term, but it became irreversibly cemented into the fluctuating nomenclature of hepatic histopathology.

A landmark in the establishment of autoimmunity as a disease process was the conference organized by the New York Academy of Sciences in 1965 (W. Dameshek, E. Witebsky, and F. Milgrom, co-chairmen) at which Dr. Popper and I shared the hepatology segment (*Ann NY Acad Sci* 1985; 124:767, 781). Dr. Popper's paper generously acknowledged that the Australian investigations had stimulated his study of immunologic components in the histogenesis of cirrhosis, and he re-emphasized piecemeal necrosis as the morphologic expression of self-perpetuation. Endorsement by Popper of any concept in hepatology was a sufficient stimulus to pursue it to the limit. Autoimmunity in liver disease became the topic of stirring debates with Hans Popper, with one of the issues being whether autoimmune hepatitis occurred *sui generis*—the mutant or forbidden clone idea—or there was an initiating cause such as virus infection, with a self-perpetuating reaction as an event secondary to this, which Popper favored.

Hans Popper, with his colleague F. Paronetto, directed his attention to the immunopathology of another enigmatic liver disease, primary biliary cirrhosis (PBC). His accurate histopathologic descriptions led to his use of the more rational term of chronic nonsuppurative cholangitis and to the now widely used staging of the disease (*Progress in Liver Diseases*, vol III 1970: 336). Also, he closely examined immunofluorescence reactions on liver sections in PBC. He reported (with Paronetto) that among the Ig-producing cells in the liver those positive for 19S globulin (IgM) outnumbered those positive for 7S (IgG). Also, studies were done by immunofluorescence on the binding of serum of patients with PBC to liver sections, showing antinuclear antibody and also an antibody to an "organ-specific" antigen, a presumed glycoprotein in proliferated biliary ductular cells, occurring only in liver diseases and in chronic ulcerative colitis (*N Engl J Med* 1964; 271: 1123). In this context, note can be taken of current identification of specific biliary glycoprotein antigens (*Proc Natl Acad Sci USA* 1988; 85:6959).

In the late 1960s, the identification of the hepatitis B surface antigen (HBsAg), and its association with hepatitis B virus (HBV) infection, in acute and in chronic hepatitis, was a major advance that Popper promoted with great vigor: he rapidly became a world reference center for "HBV-ology." I recall one of our lively coffee-table discussions, during a meeting on hepatitis in Toronto (*Can Med Assoc J* 1972; 106:417–528), which led us to a novel hypothesis in which the major types of chronic hepatitis had the same origin, the hepatitis B virus, with the host response dictating the type of outcome. A deficient immune response to the virus resulted in its persistence, associated with hepatocellular damage, a normal response resulted in elimination, and an unregulated response to host components incorporated in the HBsAg particle resulted in a chronic autoimmune reaction. The hypothesis (*Lancet* 1972; 1:1161) was only partly right, since later studies in Melbourne showed that most cases of autoimmune hepatitis, from various countries of origin, were free of all markers of infection with HBV. Of course, it is not excluded that another virus (or viruses) will fulfill the postulated initiating role in autoimmune hepatitis. One notes in passing that, even after some 30 years, there is still no accepted formulation for the origin or mechanism(s) of liver cell damage in autoimmune hepatitis. If only Hans Popper could be recalled for a fresh look at the question!

Before leaving chronic hepatitis, a note of admiration could be directed toward the role of Hans Popper in the deliberations of the "international group" of pathologists which, in a number of meeting reports (*Lancet* 1968; 2:626, 1971; 1:333, and 1977; 2:914) did so much to rationalize concepts and terminology of chronic hepatitis. The differentiation of chronic active from chronic persistent hepatitis is critically relevant to pathogenesis, and the development of consensus statements on histopathology were surely stimulated by Popper's analytical perceptions through the microscope. His other major contribution to international consensus was his membership in the Criteria Committee and Editing Board, with Carroll M. Leevy and Sheila Sherlock, of the Fogarty International Center Proceedings No. 22, "Diseases of the Liver and Biliary Tract: Standardization of Nomenclature, Diagnostic Criteria and Diagnostic Methodology," published in 1976.

Hepatocellular cancer (HCC) was always high on the list of Popper's interests and insights, and his many contributions covered human disease and the animal models. These contributions ranged from morphological description to analysis of causal processes, including HBV in man and the animal hosts of hepadna viruses, and chemicals in the case of liver cancer induced by chemical carcinogenic compounds in rodents. I was given the responsibility in 1981 as meeting secretary and co-editor, with K. Okuda, for a UICC monograph on hepatocellular cancer. The editors' tasks were greatly alleviated by a highly talented workshop panel, among whom Hans Popper stood out. This was by reason of his authoritative perspectives on every facet of hepatocellular carcinoma, derived either from his first-hand research knowledge or his command of the literature. Popper's ideas permeated into all sections of the Report (UICC Technical Report Series 74) whether the discussion was on the histopathological classifications of HCC, the geo-epidemiology of HCC, the nature and evolution of nodules induced by carcinogenic chemicals, the significance of oval cells as reparative stem cells or oncogenic markers, or the role of molecular genomic integration of hepatitis B virus.

Passing years in no way blunted Hans Popper's creativity or capacity for novel ideas. My last personal memoir would be his encouragement to consider the deficiencies of the aging liver (*Progress in Liver Diseases*, vol 8 1986:659). His statements on hepatologic problems in aging (*Aging in Liver and Gastrointestinal Tract*, L. Bianchi, et al., eds., 1987:383) epitomize his latter-day style and, above all, illustrate his extraordinary depth of knowledge of contemporary biology, liver-related and otherwise. As an overview of aging in general, this conspectus could scarcely be bettered. Among the many points of interest emphasized therein was the long life span of hepatocytes with only a few mitoses during their entire life—seemingly about three. If this is so, theories of aging that depend on the accumulation of DNA error mutations during cell replication might not seem applicable to the liver. Dr. Popper's reflections did not consider a novel idea that is of much interest to present colleagues of mine, that mutations of mitochondrial DNA, with failure of energy-producing enzyme systems, might be applicable to aging in various tissues (*Lancet* 1989; 1:642). We would have dearly liked to have had Hans Popper's response to this notion, with the liver as a particular example.

25

R.N.M. MacSween and M.P. MacSween, Glasgow

Hans Popper visited us on two occasions in Glasgow. On his first visit in 1978, he spent 2 days in the department. I remember having a long and animated discussion with him on his first morning; he, complete with pad and pencil, making a few notes. Then he said, "Now could I please meet the younger members of the staff." Of course, I was delighted that I should have the honor to introduce him around the department and allow him to discuss the research of the junior staff members, but I remember reflecting initially: "Roddy, maybe you're getting old." Then I realized that there was no younger and more alert mind than Hans'.

He had agreed to give a slide seminar in the afternoon and indicated he did not want to have a preview of the slides, preferring to deal with each case *ex tempore*. The first slide, a cirrhotic liver, was projected and I indicated this was from a 14-year-old boy. "No! No! please tell me nothing—now I know the diagnosis!" He did, of course; he was not being pedantic, however, but wanted to emphasize to us all that the pathologist should always be objective in his assessment of histological material.

His second visit in 1982 (see Fig. 20 in photo section) was as a member of the "gnomes," and Marjory has been largely responsible for the following ode in which reference is made to some of those qualities that endeared Hans to us all.

Scottish Ode to an Honoured Gnome

To the "gnomes" of Zurich, Hans was the best
So full of wisdom, wit and zest.

The group, a jigsaw from far and near,
But only complete when Hans was there.
Whether in Leuven, Vienna, or Basel,
Washington, New York, or Kassel
Hans Popper came to put his view
Awarding praise where such was due,
His spoken English somewhat flat in
He claimed fluency only in Latin!

It was never wise to sleep next door
For Hans did press ups on the floor,
Very early in the morning
The thumping coming as a warning;
For lesser "gnomes," 'twas time to rise
The day might hold some new surprise
Each "gnome" happy to acknowledge
He'd learn more this week, than a year in college.

And later, always full of charm
He'd walk the ladies arm in arm
To concert, theatre, or dinner
We ladies thought him quite a stunner.
At dinner parties midst food and drinks
He'd nod off, smiling, for 40 winks.
Refreshed, he'd take up where he'd broken
As though he'd heard each word we'd spoken.

The "gnomes" came to Glasgow in '82
We welcomed Hans and Lina too.
We sailed Loch Lomond by calm moonlight
Sipping malts to our hearts delight
To the Castle gun-room there to dine
With haggis, cranachan, and wine.

As "gnomes" the group is well selected
From Mallory bodies in liver protected.
We also self induce enzymes
To counteract the super times
We've spent in every gnomish haven
Since first we met in '67.

Hans, influential seeds you'd sown
And large oaks from small acorns grown.
We know in years that lie ahead
We'll recall the many things you said.
The "gnomes" group will stay alert and free
Honoring your memory.

26

Reba Kasten Nosoff, New York

HANS POPPER, PRESIDENT AND DEAN

SUNDAY, MARCH 19, 1972 It was a lovely Sunday, early afternoon, when the phone rang. "Reba, Dr. Popper here. Dr. James [Mount Sinai's president and dean] died today. Can you come right away to my office? We have to notify the chairmen." My heart sank. I couldn't believe what I'd heard. Come to Dr. Popper's office? It was significant that he "took charge" of this terrible situation in his Atran Building office—his home-away-from-home as we later learned.

I had always heard of Dr. Popper, for he was a legend in his own time. As chairman of the Department of Pathology (see Fig. 21 in photo section), he had brought it to new heights, and his reputation in liver diseases was already internationally known. He loved Mount Sinai, and when he saw that the hospital would have inferior residents without a medical school, he set about trying to rectify the situation. But the trustees had to be persuaded, and they were quite content with what they knew was a superior hospital. Ah, but which of us could ever resist the Dr. Popper who had made a decision about what was best for us? A committee was formed, a modest amount of money committed to looking into the formation of a medical school, and consequently The Mount Sinai School of Medicine was born. (I'm passing over the anguish and pain that went into the planning process, but Dr. Popper was certain his course was the right one.)

Dr. Popper became the first dean for academic affairs, and it was after I became the assistant to Dr. James, the first president and dean, that I came to know Dr. Popper better—but not well. He was a strong force behind the scenes and a man everyone wanted on their side.

I arrived in Dr. Popper's office, Atran 4, on that March Sunday and found others there, but I was so overcome with sadness myself I can't remember who they were. I *do* remember Dr. Popper, however. His face showed deep concern and sadness, but he was guiding us with strength and assurance that everything would work out (somehow). Gustave L. Levy, chairman of the board of trustees at that time, asked Dr. Popper to be acting president and dean while the search committee began its work, and he accepted: not with enthusiasm, but with full assurance that, in fact, no one could do it better than he; thus, the two of us began working together.

At first, suddenly filled with timidity, he would not sit at the president's desk, preferring to sit at the table to work. Gradually, he moved to the desk, where he soon appeared to have always been. He believed that Mount Sinai should have more scientists in the Academy of Sciences, and he encouraged young people to engage in research whenever he had the opportunity. It was also a sadness to him that he was invited to speak all over the world, but Mount Sinai rarely used him for teaching. He wanted Mount Sinai to become a center in liver diseases, and to that end he convinced his good friend, Dr. Henry Stratton, to establish the Stratton Liver Fund.

He wanted to keep the trustees informed and truly looked to Mr. Levy for guidance. He would write a letter to him every Friday, and Mr. Levy would give his answers and opinions on the letter and send it back immediately. (Those letters are now in the Mount Sinai archives.) If there was disagreement, a phone conversation ensued. Dr. Popper liked Mr. Levy's succinct efficiency. Mr. Levy admired Dr. Popper.

Dr. Popper instituted some strict rules as interim president and dean. The word "retired" was to be stricken from our vocabulary. He was *not* retired, and he wanted everyone in the scientific community to be aware of that fact. He did not have to worry on that score. He was one of the most prolific scientists ever, and his colleagues at the NIH once told us that a month never passed without something new and important from Dr. Popper. No one was to call him by his first name—and hardly anyone ever did, except Gus Levy and some of the trustees. This small rule commanded a respect that evaporated with the use of first names, and he knew this.

He did not want to mix his liver diseases work with his dean's work. He put in a full day in the dean's office (Guggenheim 8), eating his yogurt lunch at his desk. At 5 p.m., he left our office and went to Atran 4, where he did what he *really* loved, and worked there until 11 p.m. When colleagues suggested he bring his microscope to the president and dean's office, he quickly rejected the idea. One had nothing to do with the other, and when he was busy with whichever office, that one had his full attention.

He believed in fair representation—but not necessarily democracy—in policies he felt were for the good of the institution. When the City University instituted a 6-year program in the biological sciences, which would guarantee a place in medical school for those in the program, each of the New York medical schools were asked to take a few students. At Mount Sinai, the chairmen formed a committee to study the curriculum and goals of this new idea, and reported back to the faculty that they felt the program was inferior and their students would not be up to the caliber of our own students. Meanwhile, Chancellor Kibbee, then in charge of the City University, informed Dr. Popper that every medical school had agreed to accept three or four, and here we were, affiliated with the City University, and refusing to accept any. The chancellor felt changes in curriculum, etc., could be ironed out later, but he saw the 6-year program as an asset for allowing bright minority students to enter medical school. Dr. Popper called a meeting of the chairmen and announced to them the agenda: "how many" students we would tell the Chancellor we accept. The chairmen broke into heated conversation. "How many?" Had they not already said they would take none? Dr. Popper remained calm. At that time, Dr. Popper's hearing was not acute, or so he said, and he often pretended not to hear this or that— even after he began to wear a hearing device. I loved his performance when he began to act as though he couldn't hear. On this day, he kept asking for a vote of how many students we should take, completely ignoring the bruhaha going on around him. Beaten down, the chairmen voted to take three or four, and Dr. Popper concluded the meeting with what someone once termed his "Mona Lisa" smile. When I later asked one of the chairmen why they acquiesced finally, he replied, "Who wants to stir Dr. Popper's ire?"

Dr. Popper's temper was a fearful trait. My office was dreadfully afraid of him when he was in one of his "tempers," but, because I spent a lot of time with him in his office, I realized he actually could turn his wrath on and off at will. On really important matters, he was cool and calm. But waiting for elevators, whether in Guggenheim or in Atran, drove him wild, and he would kick them with such force, I'm sure they secretly groaned. There were certain people whose voices on the phone would raise his temperature to boiling.

His own work habits were so efficient and organized, he had no patience for anyone who seemed to yield under pressure. Our office had an enormous amount of work to do in addition to the work Dr. Popper generated. When he would come out to the secretaries and ask if they had done something he wanted, if the answer was not an immediate "yes," he would declare they were unable to do it and he would "take it home to Lina" to do. No, no, the secretaries would cry out. They would do it right away. Poor Lina; we all knew she had a full-time job just being Mrs. Popper. We also knew he thought nothing of calling her at 3:30 p.m. to tell her he had visitors from Europe he was bringing home for dinner. I often wondered how she ever got a dinner together on such short notice. She never complained, and Dr. Popper made no bones about the fact that he absolutely adored her. If we were unsure about an invitation for something, or a menu, anything at all—he would say, "I'll ask Lina," and he did. The next day we would have her opinion.

I loved working on papers with him, because he was a wonderful storyteller, and something he would be putting in his paper would remind him of a happening in his past. Gradually, I began putting his unbelievable past together and to understand the difficulties he encountered on his way to his present notoriety. We shared authorship on two papers, and it was one of the greatest honors he could have bestowed. Writing for Dr. James was easy. Writing with Dr. Popper was so difficult. I would take home some of his former writings so I could understand his ideas and philosophy. He was a true medical intellectual, never satisfied with someone else's results, always seeking his own answers and then joyously sharing them with others. He loved teaching young people. In his older years, he would say he needed young people around the world to be his eyes in the microscope, since his own were not so strong anymore: but *he* would have to tell them what to look for, since their knowledge was not yet in full bloom. And they did just that. Scientists all over the world called or came to him to show him slides they felt were interesting, or to ask his opinion, or just to learn from him.

Gradually, my office staff grew to love him, and when the search committee at last came up with a successor (Dr. Chalmers—the suggestion that Dr. Chalmers be considered came from Dr. Popper) we were sorry to see him go back to Atran. The trustees and the search committee talked with Dr. Popper about his accepting the job full-time, but he said he was too old. Yet, his ideas were always young, and had he remained in that position, we would have done something new and innovative with the curriculum, which would have startled the medical school world and perhaps changed the course of teaching, for he was not afraid to try some daring idea, nor did he fear admitting failure and trying something else.

When Dr. Selikoff invited Dr. Popper to become a part of their environmental sciences division of community medicine, he felt this was "soft science," about which he knew very little. Before long, however, he was wrapped up in whether or not the environment affected the liver, if at all, and the effects of Agent Orange on the liver.

Later, when the Department of Geriatrics was opened under the leadership of Dr. Robert Butler, Dr. Popper was asked to become interested in and work with aging problems. It was during that period that Dr. Popper very excitedly told us one day that he had discovered livers don't age. Therefore, the transplant opportunities were endless. He grew determined that Mount Sinai should be in the vanguard of liver transplants in New York and masterminded the idea of a consortium with other hospitals. But he did not have the pleasure of witnessing the successful liver transplant program now in effect at Mount Sinai.

Dr. Popper was an impeccable dresser. He was an avid exerciser and thus was very strong. From time to time a bright colored shirt or sweater would appear, and, when we would compliment him, he would say, "Lina picked it out. What do I know?" By the same token, he noticed everything about the women in the office, often commenting on how nice they looked or that he liked a new hairstyle. They never had anyone before or after him who did that.

At the first commencement over which Dr. Popper presided, he asked my advice about which of his 12 or so honorary degrees he should wear on his robe. He brought some for me to look at, and I thought the ermine tails on his degree from Bologna had panache. You will see that particular award on the shoulder of his academic robes in the various pictures of those occasions (see Fig. 22 in photo section). He looked very grand. After he no longer served as dean, he refused the invitation to be grand marshall at the commencement exercises saying that honor was for "old people."

Although Dr. Popper had "stage fright" before presiding over an investiture or commencement, or even his own symposia for that matter, he was in full command once they began, and he loved the parties afterward. He was always "stuck" on the dais, he complained, and would leap down when he felt the urge to dance, swooping up one or another of the ladies. He and Janet Levy used to have an especially good time on the dance floor. Dr. Popper was a good dancer, even though he always wore rubber-soled shoes.

After Dr. Popper turned the president and dean role over to Dr. Chalmers (Fig. 23), he rarely came back to our office. He never wanted Dr. Chalmers to feel he was being critical or offering suggestions, or spying. If anyone wanted to see him, they could always find him in Atran in the evenings, and everyone at some time or another went down there to consult with him.

However, he and I remained friends forever, and sometimes he would honor me by calling and asking *my* opinion on something (Fig. 24). He would always call before going on a trip to let me know where he and Lina would be and how long they would be gone. Then I would receive a postcard from him and Lina, and signatures of all his colleagues he worked with—Dr. Sheila Sherlock, Dr. Gerber, Dr. Falk, etc. I still have those cards.

He and Dr. Chalmers shared similar birth dates, so I would celebrate with both at dinner in my home (Figs. 25 and 26) together with some of their friends, such as the Butlers and the Salans. Dr. Popper loved cream puffs, and I would bake an abundance of those for him. Poor Dr. Chalmers got cream puffs in lieu of a birthday cake whether he liked them or not.

When I left Mount Sinai, over Dr. Popper's protestations, he would call every week, sometimes on a Sunday afternoon from his laboratory, to see what was new; we would compare Columbia-Presbyterian (where I am now) with Mount Sinai, he would tell me what was new with him, we would quarrel about politics (he was *not* a liberal), and we would talk (gossip a little?) about folks we knew.

As a farewell present when Dr. Popper left the president's office, we gave him a gold heart with the words "Remember Us." As luck would have it, the jeweler mistakenly wrote "Remember U.S." What would Dr. Popper think we were trying to tell him? In desperation, we tried to have the periods removed quickly because we wanted to present it to him. The period removal was not completely successful, but we presented him with the "defective" heart anyhow, telling him what had happened. His face was bright with pleasure, and he mounted it on a piece of velvet, framed it, and hung it in his office.

When I visit Lina Popper, and we sit in Dr. Popper's study talking, I've noticed she has that little framed heart on display with some of his other things. It is questionable whether he really remembered us, I suppose, but I can tell you that we—and certainly I—will never forget him.

27

Kunio Okuda, Chiba

It was in 1975, if I recall correctly, that I first introduced myself to Hans by asking for a foreword to my monograph entitled, *Radiological Aspects of the Liver and Biliary Tract: X-Ray and Radioisotope Diagnosis,* to be published by Igaku-Shoin, Tokyo/Year Book, Chicago. I was not certain about his response, thinking that he would either refuse my request or respond only minimally, because he was not a clinician and was more interested in histopathology. To my delight, he gave me a great foreword I really did not deserve, in which he even said to the effect that gross diagnosis, if it advances and becomes accurate, would obviate the necessity for histological diagnosis that requires invasive biopsy. I, then, met him in person in Pécs, Hungary, on the occasion of the meeting of the International Association for the Study of the Liver (IASL); he had been looking for me when I arrived. I still remember this meeting vividly. He was sitting in the front row in the hall and waiting for the opening of the session. His paper was the first one, and he appeared so impatient. No sooner was he called upon than he jumped to the podium and presented his study on vinyl-chloride-induced Banti's syndrome and angiosarcoma. He had since been very helpful, like a father, to me by giving appropriate suggestions, new information, ideas, and philosophy. He was so honest, unassuming, and he always told me frankly what he knew, what he did not, and what he really thought. He had made a great impact and influence on my thinking as a hepatologist/scientist. The European history as told by him was so fascinating that I thought he could have been a historian.

I regret that on many occasions I disappointed him, the person who recommended me and made me the president of IASL in 1978, by not living up to his expectations. In that year, in a postgraduate course held in Madrid, he told me that I should not have given the talk from the manuscript. I was aware, but due to the language difficulty, that was what I did. I reflected that I should have taken time and memorized the talk so that I did not need a manuscript. Sometimes his English was a consolation to me, whose English pronunciation is just as bad as his. Amazingly, people tried hard to understand his English, which I also had difficulty in understanding. It took me quite some time to get used to it. Some Americans said to me that my English was just as difficult to understand as Hans'. The only difference has been that people do not try to understand me.

I often wondered how he kept all the information and references well sorted out; he was very well versed with the current and past publications. At meetings, he often told me about certain papers or a book that would interest me, and he always kept his word by sending them to me after his return to New York. He was fair and unbiased in assessing scientific work, although he was critical and was always excited with new findings, which he would pass along to me. I learned a great deal from him not only about science, but philosophy as well. He always sought international leadership in hepatology, and indeed he kept it throughout despite his age. He once said to me that to serve as an editor for a journal is an important scientific contribution, but that an editor makes only enemies, no friends. I am currently experiencing this phenomenon myself!

In his last several years, he was particularly interested in hepatocarcinogenesis. He went to Alaska and studied hepatocellular carcinoma among Eskimos who were not cirrhotic. He told me that it was somewhat similar to woodchuck hepatocellular carcinoma and paid attention to inflammation around the mass. He sent me a draft of his paper in which he emphasized necroinflammation as the change of etiologic significance in malignant transformation. I was not quite convinced and asked for the tissue slides on which he based his idea. He was kind enough to send them to me. He always sought truth and was open-minded, listening to opinions of others, even objections. The last time I was with him was in Chicago during the AASLD meeting. He wanted to talk with me and we sat at a table for more than an hour. He must have anticipated his approaching death. He talked of various things to me in earnest. He confessed to me that he made a big mistake when he emphasized piecemeal necrosis as the change leading to cirrhosis; having heard in pursuing years various clinical reports, he now believed that chronic liver disease progressed to cirrhosis by means of repeated flare-ups, not continuously by piecemeal necrosis.

Toward the end of his life, he kept writing to me of the pain he was experiencing and his clinical condition. It was heart-breaking that I could not help him at all even though he trusted me as a clinician.

On the personal side, I particularly liked him as a person and a friend. He was very sociable and liked to drink and meet and chat with people. Lina and Hans came to Chiba at least three times, and I have a number of fond recollections. Once we took Lina, Hans, and a few American friends to a scenic spot at the tip of Boso Peninsula and had a geisha party. He liked Japanese sake just as he did geishas. There was a show in the hotel basement, and he insisted on going despite opposition from Lina. We all danced and had fun. Hinae, my wife, told me later that Hans had very strong muscles as evidenced by the strength with which he held his partners. One evening, we went to a Japanese style restaurant and he had to remove his shoes. Hinae noted that his sock had a small hole. He was a person who did not bother with nonscientific things, but it reminded me of the days when we were under American occupation. He did, indeed, serve in the U.S. Army in Japan at that time, as I understand. American soldiers used to be invited to Japanese homes and were embarrassed when asked to take off their shoes; socks had holes that we used to call "potatoes." Soon came the era of nylon fabrics, and two things became strong after World War II in Japan: women and socks! During the last war, cloth material became scarce, and poor synthetic fabrics called "sufu" in Japanese were used for making socks that easily wore out. Nylon introduced a significant change in durability of socks. On another occasion, when he was invited by Prof. Nakashima, Kurume University, I had the honor of accompanying his party to a hot spring resort called "Unzen." We all stayed in a Japanese-style hotel. Early in the morning, we heard noise coming from his room lasting for quite some time. At breakfast, he told us that he was practicing American soldiers' pushups, his regular prebreakfast exercise. No wonder he was always physically fit and had strong arms. In 1982, when I was the president of the Asian-Pacific Association for the Study of the Liver and organized the scientific meeting in Hong Kong, Lina and Hans were among the invitees. The meeting was followed by a postgraduate course organized by Prof. Chung in Seoul, Korea. All liver dignitaries were invited. In Seoul, the boys had fun at night at a stag party, where a fair companion sits next to you and feeds you like a mother bird does her baby birds. Sheila insisted on joining the men. Poor Sheila, she could not sit still when Gerry cheek-danced with a beautiful Kesen geisha. Hans developed diarrhea there. Subsequently, he had to give a lecture in Tokyo. Hinae met his party in Narita and brought them to Tokyo just in time for the evening reception. He did not look well. Two days later, he confided in me that he felt so bad at Jikei University

Hospital where he lectured, because this old hospital did not have western-style comfort facilities, it had only the old Japanese toilet, and he had not trained his legs strong enough to use it. He trained his arms by doing pushups, but not his legs.

There are many fond memories of him; fortunately, I have photos of the many events at which we were together. I miss him so much, but he lives on in my mind.

28

Fiorenzo Paronetto, New York
Nijole Brazenas, Yonkers

"WER IMMER STREBEND SICH BEMÜHT, DEN KÖNNEN WIR ERLÖSEN."
"WHOEVER ASPIRING, STRUGGLES ON,
FOR HIM THERE IS SALVATION."

Goethe, "Faust," quoted by H. Popper

It is more than 3 years since Dr. Popper's death, and our memory of him is still unchanged with time. Others may remember him as a founder of a medical school, a visionary dean, a catalyst of several national and international groups, and a successful researcher, but for us he will be remembered mostly as a stimulating teacher and a friend.

The two of us came to Mount Sinai Hospital in July 1957 from different lands. One of us arrived from his native Italy with the aim to initiate a career in pathology and research. During his previous visit, he was a pupil of Dr. David Adlersberg, a Viennese physician, who introduced him to the frustrations and joys of research and was responsible for his returning to the United States. Dr. Adlersberg suggested that he should continue his research with his friend, Dr. Popper, a Viennese pathologist who had just left Cook County Hospital in Chicago to join Mount Sinai Hospital. In the 1950s, research opportunities in Italy were practically nonexistent and a young scientist needed encouragement, stimulation, and opportunities to follow the hypotheses of one's work. Dr. Popper has both stimulated research and provided the tools to perform meaningful research.

The other pupil of Dr. Popper arrived in the United States from Lithuania through refugee camps in Austria, where she had graduated from Medical School in Innsbruck and had been fortunate to be accepted in Mount Sinai Hospital's pathology residency program.

We remember July 1, 1957, when we, with 17 other residents, convened in the residents' room in the first floor of the Atran Building to meet our new chairman. As was his style, Dr. Popper began to pace the room. After welcoming us, he reminded us that we were there to start together a most enjoyable time of our lives dedicated only to learning. He added:

> Experience is a major asset that augments with time. While in other fields, like physics and mathematics, the peak of achievements is in the second or third decade; in pathology the maximum performance increases with age. We should not therefore waste time; that is the most precious commodity we have.

He emphasized that our energies should be geared toward becoming "complete pathologists," physicians who should excel in all three facets of pathology: diagnosis, teaching, and research. He told us:

> Pathology is a discipline that has firm roots both in basic and clinical sciences. It is an undivided discipline with three intertwined areas of teaching, research, and diagnostic pathology. Each member of the department of pathology should be a teacher, diagnostician, and researcher. Deep knowledge in these three fields can be obtained only through subspecialization because it is impossible to master all fields of pathology. "Research in pathology is important. It focuses traditionally on the development of new knowledge about the causes and mechanisms of human diseases utilizing all available techniques. Thus, research in pathology is a bridge between basic and clinical biomedical sciences, a quest for knowledge about the pathogenesis of diseases, knowledge that can lead to new diagnostic tools, prognostic insights, and rational therapy.

In the 30 years that followed, he remained faithful to his credo and was a role model for all of us.

Dr. Popper's love for pathology and teaching became apparent during the years of our residency in pathology. As a teacher he always cherished the signout conferences with the residents. His daily signout conferences, which more officially were performed on Saturdays with the participation of the entire senior staff, were the center of our activities. Promptly at 9 a.m. the conference room was filled with residents. They projected the histological slides, and this was followed by a soliloquy by Dr. Popper on the pathogenesis of the lesions presented. This showed his encyclopedic knowledge of all fields of pathology. It was frequently interspersed with stories about his Viennese career and Viennese physicians and teachers: Rokitansky, who first described the acute yellow atrophy; Eppinger, who first characterized catarrhal jaundice, what we now call viral hepatitis; and Hering, who first illustrated the connecting link between bile canaliculi and ductules.

The "organ recital," the review of the weekly autopsies, embodied the old dictum originated in the Morgagni amphitheater in Bologna, which he displayed in the autopsy room: "Hic locus est ubi mors gaudet succurrere vitae," that is, "this is the place where death is glad to help life." He enjoyed the exercise to reconstruct from the observation of the organs the clinical history of the patients.

He was particularly happy when from the keen observation of the organs he could correctly identify the original disease. "Autopsies are our great teachers," he used to say. "There are no uninteresting routine autopsies, only routine pathologists." The weekly CPC's (clinical pathological conferences), his most cherished teaching exercises, enabled him to utilize his gift for correlating and illustrating various disease entities. He occasionally enjoyed switching roles to discuss as a clinician the cases to be presented; confirmation of his ability as a clinician that reminded him of the times he practiced internal medicine, hepatology, and endocrinology in Vienna. The fame of the CPCs went beyond the walls of our institution, and CPCs were repeated in various national and international meetings. He used to say that the preparation of the CPC was a particularly rewarding experience because he could always learn new facets of the protean manifestations of pathology.

A particular pleasure came to him during the Monday night research meetings. Here all the staff involved in various research activities would meet, discuss the data, and prepare the plan for the week. We remember his ability in gathering the data and making sense of often uninterpretable results. Those were the times when he became interested in the pathogenesis of fibrosis, ductular cell proliferation, and the development of nodules and tumors in animals undergoing treatment with various carcinogens.

We remember some tragicomic and painful moments. The beginning of the meetings in 1957 was ill-starred because many valuable rats in prolonged ethionine diet shipped from his previous laboratory in Chicago had escaped from the cages during the flight and had joined the untreated control animals. This mishap had delayed the initiation of experiments for several months. A painful ordeal was usually experienced in preparation for the annual pathology meetings when the senior authors would present their papers that frequently were torn apart so that the humbled presenter had to start anew.

As a researcher, he instilled in us the curiosity to investigate the causes and mechanisms of human diseases utilizing rigorous morphological examination supported by all available techniques. He advised us to formulate only testable hypotheses because nontestable hypotheses or questions that may lead to more than one answer are not worth pursuing; to ask only the important questions, because often it takes the same time to solve both significant and trivial problems; and be loyal to collaborators because they forge our thoughts and knowledge.

He used to repeat that it is easy to have ideas, but it is difficult to persevere with the accepted idea. One does not need fancy equipment or sophisticated reagents to collect important data: the hematoxylin and eosin stain is sufficient for the thinking mind. Research should be done with the buttocks: sitting long hours at the microscope.

Writing a paper with Dr. Popper was an unusual experience. Here the entire personality of Dr. Popper could be savored: his restless pacing back and forth through his office, his boundless energy, his rapid association of different facts, his tremendous memory for the bibliography that, in his precomputer age, enabled him to retrieve rapidly reprints and bibliographic data, his painful editing and re-editing until the paper met his high standards. "A paper is ready to be sent for publication," he used to say, "when you went over it so many times that, rereading again, you feel nauseated." He was very loyal to his collaborators, and he would always finish a paper, often only out of a feeling of duty and loyalty.

For us, the research in the Department of Pathology is enshrined with tender memories. It is during the gathering of data and writing of a paper on the hepatic effects of carrageenan—a seaweed that stimulates fibrosis—that the two of us, both residents in pathology, met and initiated the courtship that continued in our lives together.

Many things changed since those years in the 1950s. With the student revolution of the 1960s, the style of Dr. Popper changed: his authoritarian, Viennese manner mellowed into a more democratic, paternalistic mood.

As a diagnostician, he was unsurpassed in reaching a correct diagnosis without the benefit of clinical data. He was a master in reconstructing the patient's clinical history from the liver biopsy—a sort of game that he enjoyed up to the last days of his life in frequent conferences at the Bronx Veterans Administration Medical Center and at the Albert Einstein Liver Center. He used to say that the study of patients' cases has been his inspiration and stimulation. In this respect, he was a real empiricist following the inductive approach of his beloved Francis Bacon—the 16th century philosopher—that man can attain truth by detailed analysis of the facts.

Later, we saw Dr. Popper less frequently; he traveled extensively, and his circle of friends and activities spanned the globe. Toward the end of his life, we treasured his renewed friendship when his disease progressively reduced his activities and directed his outlook more toward the past and the future than the present.

He would then frequently discuss the scope of pathology in academic institutions. He was convinced that pathology was in decline because pathologists had not followed their primary vocation: diagnosis, teaching, and research of the pathogenesis of human diseases. The mission of academic pathology is to train pathologists who can effectively apply the emerging technologies to diagnostic pathology and interpret the results scientifically. He would always welcome with joy his collaborators and friends, but he was always seeking new knowledge. He would frequently say: "Tell me what is new about the liver, not about politics. At my age, I have to retain only necessary information. Because of my daily loss of neurons each new information will displace an older one."

When we advanced in age and maturity, he became a friend, revealing a more human aspect of himself. At this time, the old memories of his native Vienna and his family would come back incessantly. He would remember with emotion the Christmas carols of Vienna that were embodied in the *Sound of Music*, his difficult years as a refugee, his hopes for the department that bears his name, his love for Lina, which always supported him during his hectic life. On his way home from work, he frequently stopped at the florist to buy some red roses for her. "I love Lina," he used to say, "and in this way I express my love and beg forgiveness for the many hours spent away from her." Never willing to let the pain of his terminal illness interfere with the work to be done, he finished his last two papers that returned to themes of his early work: "Viral Versus Chemical Carcinogenesis" and "The Relation of Mesenchymal Cell Products to the Bile Ductular System."

When he sent off his last paper, conscious of the severity of his illness, he said, "I do not have time to wait for the reviewer and to answer the critiques. I will send the manuscript to my friend Dame Sheila Sherlock. She will take care of this work." He then cleaned his desk of all scientific papers: it was almost as if he was saying goodbye to a group of old friends. "I wish that my work will not be forgotten and will continue in the hands of my pupils: viral and chemical carcinogenesis . . . ductular cell proliferation. . . ." We had restarted each Saturday, like in the old times, to review at the microscope livers of the woodchucks that would develop tumors after injection of the woodchuck hepatitis virus—a virus that closely resembles human hepatitis virus. He had predicted that this experimental model would be the key to unraveling the pathogenesis of tumors induced by viruses or chemicals. He was fighting against pain and drowsiness, and he would often fall asleep while looking through the microscope.

The last time he looked in the microscope he was going over a most unusual liver slide with the spectrum of preneoplastic and neoplastic liver lesions in a woodchuck that had been treated with a chemical carcinogen. "These findings are so beautiful—he exclaimed—I will take some pictures . . . but now I am so tired. . . . We will take the pictures next time."

But there was not to be a next time. Dr. Popper was admitted to the hospital and he died shortly thereafter. A great pathologist is now enshrined in our memories: a diagnostician, a teacher, a researcher, and a friend who conferred on us a legacy that we will always cherish.

29

Victor Perez, *Buenos Aires*

I spent 1958 and 1959 working with Hans Popper. After that, even if we were separated by 10,000 kilometers, we saw each other at least once a year, in New York or someplace in the world where a liver meeting was taking place. I will try to recall situations of those years that remain in my memory.

I started to work with Hans at the beginning of January 1958. He had just moved from Chicago and was trying to organize the Department of Pathology at Mount Sinai Hospital in New York. Fenton Schaffner was still in Chicago and arrived a few months later. At this time, I was trained in gastroenterology and had little experience in pathology.

On my first day at work, Hans was very busy and, to get rid of me, he gave me a couple of dark boxes full of slides and sent me to a microscope in the corner of the last room of the department. For a couple of weeks, I spent all my time studying liver biopsies. The only person I talked to was Humi, a young Japanese technician, who was a survivor of the Hiroshima bombing.

One day, all of a sudden, Hans dropped in at my little place. He took me to his desk and showed me a few liver biopsies he had received in consultation from different places in the country and from abroad. This moment was, for me, the beginning of a very productive and inspiring association. We used to review the material on Saturdays and also on Sundays. Sometimes we had a break and walked together along Madison Avenue to a nearby fruit store owned by an Italian family. Hans used to ask for peaches and grapes, speaking a funny Italian.

My first publication while at Mount Sinai was a real gift from Hans. He was reviewing biopsies and necropsies from cases of hepatitis due to

Marsilid intake. The drug was in jeopardy at this time because it gave severe reactions. At Mount Sinai, there were nine cases of adverse reactions, most of them fatal. He introduced me to a resident in cardiology, Melvin Kahn, who reviewed the clinical histories. I studied the liver pathology, and we rushed to publish the cases in the famous green journal (*American Journal of Medicine* 1958; 24:898–916.

The arrival of Fenton Schaffner was very important for all of us. We started to make rounds in the clinical wards, and we discussed the most important liver cases. Then we reviewed the liver biopsies with Hans in pathology. This training in clinicopathologic correlation was, for me, most useful in the years to come.

In May 1958, a young Italian, Giorgio Menghini from Perugia, visited our laboratory. He brought a new needle for liver biopsies. Hans helped him to make his needle known in the United States, and I went with Giorgio to different hospitals, where he demonstrated his new wonder. In the same month, the World Congress of Gastroenterology took place in Washington. Hans invited me to a luncheon at the Sheraton Hotel. We were about 20 people from different countries. During this luncheon, Hans founded the International Association for the Study of the Liver.

We used to go once a month to the Department of Pathology at the Veterans Administration Hospital in the Bronx. Usually we had a quick lunch at the cafeteria and rushed to arrive for the meeting, which took place at 2 p.m. At the beginning, he drove his car. His driving was so shaky that I managed to convince him to let me go with my car. Once at the Veterans Hospital, we were received by Dr. Gordon and his staff. In a small room, we attended the routine clinical presentation by a resident followed by the description of the liver pathology. Hans appeared to doze off during the presentation. I was very embarrassed, but, to my surprise, he usually awoke and started to discuss the case very naturally. Years later, in a round table he chaired in Sao Paolo, Brazil, after an abundant lunch with wine, he slept during all the presentations, including mine. Nevertheless, when his turn arrived, he managed to summarize all the ideas and discuss the more conflicting points of the subject.

Once a week we had a research meeting in the lecture room. We started at 5 p.m. and we used to finish around 11 p.m. You would hear Japanese, Hungarian, German, Italian, and Latino-American accents. The only people who sounded unusual were the few Americans. We were interested at that time in the mechanism of fibrosis. Hans theorized that liver damage was capable of producing fibrosis without the presence of fibroblasts. With Fiorenzo Paronetto I was asked to review staining in liver biopsies, from animals as well as from humans. We published our results in the *Archives of*

Pathology (1960; 70:300) and *Laboratory Investigations* (1961; 10:265–90).

Hans pushed Fenton and me to apply electron microscopy to liver pathology. At this time, electron microscopy was an extremely sophisticated tool seldom used in liver biopsies. We devoted quite a lot of time to ultrastructural studies of liver because all liver biopsies were processed for electron microscopy. One of the very first observations made with Fenton Schaffner was the alterations in bile canaliculi in cases of jaundice due to norethandrolone. This work was published in the *Journal of Laboratory and Clinical Medicine* (1960; 56:623–8).

Hans traveled often. After each trip, he always brought new ideas and relayed histories of the interesting people he met. Sometimes he made a kind of olympic game of his trip. One evening in 1966, we met at a cocktail party in the Parque del Retiro in Madrid at 8 p.m. The same day he had given a talk in Istanbul, Turkey. In the early afternoon, on the way to Spain, he had stopped in Greece and had given a lecture in Athens.

I always admired how Hans was able to keep up to date with progress. In the 1960s, he was using pure morphology with some histochemistry. In the 1980s (and also in his 80s), he was able to summarize complicated symposia on subjects of molecular biology.

I owe a lot to Hans for his friendship through all these years and for his generosity and his continuous intellectual challenge.

30

Lawrie W. Powell,
W. Graham E. Cooksley,
and June W. Halliday,

Brisbane

Unlike many hepatologists from the United States and Europe, Hans Popper visited Australia only once in his long lifetime, but he left an indelible imprint on a large number of people.

With his continuing interest in the inauguration of societies for the study of liver disease, Hans accepted an invitation to attend the inaugural meeting of the Asian-Pacific Association for the Study of the Liver (APASL) in Auckland, New Zealand, in January 1980 and to visit some Australian centers afterwards. From the moment he and Lina set foot on New Zealand soil and encountered a Maori welcome, they became engrossed in these countries, their culture, science, and people. Throughout the APASL meeting, Hans sat in the front row, as was his custom, and regularly made constructive comments on the presentations, frequently speculating incisively well beyond what others considered the data would allow. Many who did not know him well were literally staggered by his stamina, dancing well into the night, sampling for the first time New Zealand and Australian wines, only to resume his seat in the front row early next morning. As the founding father of both the IASL and the AASLD, his suggestions and advice to the Inaugural Executive Committee were invaluable and ensured the future success of the APASL. The original constitution has remained intact since.

By the time Hans reached Australia, he was in top gear, having fully

123

recovered from jetlag. In every center that he visited, he displayed the same qualities of intellect and character for which he had been admired by Australians abroad. He had the uncanny ability to get directly to the core of a clinical problem with a succinct summary of the clinical and pathological presentations (often better summarized than by the presenters themselves) and displaying an encyclopedic knowledge of the published literature. In Brisbane, Hans was one of the most memorable guest speakers at medical grand rounds that we have witnessed. The case for discussion was a young woman with chronic hepatitis. Just before the meeting began, Hans was invited to review the histological slides of the case. After doing so briefly, he announced to the bewildered hosts that he needed to visit his room at the hospital VIP flat before the meeting! This request was duly complied with and the meeting began 5 minutes late. At the appropriate time during Hans' discussion of the histology of the case, he produced a series of highly relevant photomicrographs including some of experimental non-A, non-B hepatitis in chimpanzees, with features very similar to the case under discussion. As usual, his discussion of the case was masterful, with a logical account of the pathobiology, differential diagnosis, and symptomatology, constantly relating the relevant published data to the clinical problem.

In every center he visited Hans actively encouraged young people, firing their interest and enthusiasm in hepatology and promoting the study of liver disease.

Australia, in turn, left its indelible imprint on Hans and Lina when they had their unforgettable encounter with the forces of nature in the tropics of Queensland. Hans had planned their brief visit to Heron Island on the Barrier Reef with typical military precision, even requesting just before he left New York that his scheduled departure from the island be by helicopter at 5 p.m. rather than at 1 p.m. (in order that he might chat for a while with New Yorker friends arriving at 1 p.m.!). Unfortunately, on the day in question, a tropical cyclone descended on the island and the 1 p.m. helicopter was the last to leave the island before the cyclone struck. All seats were occupied and the pilot was not going to break any official rules! However, after a lively discussion between Hans and the pilot that only Lina could describe and probably understand, the pilot conceded that his vacant co-pilot's seat could be used, and, of course, Lina insisted that Hans take it. The pilot reassured Lina that she would be on the next helicopter to leave the island and she was—3 days and a tropical cyclone later! During the great "blow," all communications to the island were cut, but fortunately for all concerned there were no major repercussions. During the 3 days, Hans fulfilled all his lecturing engagements and Lina and Hans finally met up in Sydney! Even this setback had its pleasant memories (for us at least). The airport manager found Hans, in his concern for Lina's safety, more than a mouthful and was so overjoyed when one of us arrived on the scene to look after Hans that he regularly upgraded our tickets thereafter.

An example of how Hans' love of his work dominated everything occurred in a walk through a subtropical rainforest near Brisbane. Lina paused to remove a leech fastened to her ankle when she saw an enormous snake, its coils lying beside the track. Its girth was that of a man's arm except for a football-sized swelling representing its last meal. Lina was rather agitated, but, not wanting to cause panic, quickly asked its species. It was pointed out that it was a magnificent example of an amethyst python. Hans, however, was unfazed and pressed on with his discussion of hepatocellular inflammation and death!

Hans Popper had much in common with Sir Macfarlane Burnet; in particular, he loved to speculate, frequently roving well beyond what could be established experimentally. To both scholars, research lacked meaning if it was not guided and stimulated by hypotheses, presented in such a form that proof, disproof, or modification should be eventually possible. For both, their hypotheses were rarely disproved outright.

Hans Popper will be remembered in Australia particularly for his genuine curiosity about biological events, his vigorous debates, his encyclopedic knowledge of the scientific literature, for his drive and enthusiasm, and for his constant encouragement of students and young scientists.

31

Robert H. Purcell, Bethesda
John L. Gerin, Rockville

For almost a decade and a half, from the early 1970s to his death, Hans Popper was a full scientific partner in our research efforts. Over that time, he also became a close friend and mentor. He never ceased to surprise us or to give new, fresh, and "young" insights to our areas of common interest.

We first became involved with Hans in 1974, because of his interest in animal models for viral hepatitis. This was, of course, only one of his multitude of interests in the field, but one that he pursued tenaciously over the years, often to the ridicule of others who thought that he should not waste his time on animals. However, he saw early on the importance of having a manipulable model of human hepatitis. When he listened to a talk at George Washington University in 1982, given by one of us on the woodchuck model of hepadnavirus infection, he immediately recognized the significance of this model in the contrasting views of virus versus chemically induced liver cancer. Thus, he was the first to bring these two opposed and somewhat hostile fields together.

Hans was a tireless worker, reading endless hundreds of histologic slides from our many studies of experimental hepatitis in chimpanzees, marmosets, and other primates and woodchucks. Always, he wanted more, often to be stained by special methods to bring out the features he sought. Dissatisfied with his own sources of histologic preparation and, by then, "retired" and without control of such facilities, he retrained a local commercial pathology laboratory in Bethesda to prepare slides exactly to his specifications. Our slide collections still contain many of the slides read and photographed by Hans. These were accompanied by detailed histologic evaluations that were enriched by his many years of experience, none of it, apparently, forgotten.

Hans was also a prolific writer (or, rather, dictator) of letters. These were rich, rewarding, and often filled with comments, suggestions for new research projects, and encouragement. Not infrequently, they contained remonstrances because we had sent too many biopsies of normal liver (e.g., safety tests of new vaccines) or because our projects were moving too slowly for his liking. Hans had a clear and rational perception of the chronic diseases from which he suffered in his later years and wanted to use the time left to him as profitably and productively as possible. This wealth of written correspondence—pathologic reports, letters, notes of encouragement and chastisement, with copies of all correspondence to each of us, and our responses to all of this—constituted an impressive bit of literature. There was our normal correspondence file and then there was a separate file of the "Popper papers."

But this was not a collaboration only by correspondence. Hans actively and personally pursued these and his many other collaborations, often grouping them into marathon days of activity. Routinely and at frequent intervals, he would visit the Washington area from New York City, sometimes at his own expense, arriving by airline shuttle to meet with the hepatology group at the National Institutes of Health for slide presentations. From there, he would proceed to the Armed Forces Institute of Pathology at the Walter Reed Medical Center for more slide presentations. After that, he would meet with the two of us, either on the NIH campus, in R.H.P.'s office or occasionally, in Jay Hoofnagle's office, or at the Rockville Laboratory, for discussions of our ongoing studies. Often, more junior members of our laboratories would join the discussions, and Hans especially enjoyed the opportunity to impress his ideas and suggested approaches on this eager group. Following these meetings, one or the other of us would arrange transportation for him back to National Airport and his return shuttle flight to New York. These would have been exhausting days for a much younger man, and, as his health became more fragile, Lina routinely accompanied him on these sojourns, exhibiting much patience and grace.

Once, Hans and Lina were attending a meeting in the Washington area when a major blizzard struck. The heavy snow brought traffic to a standstill and paralyzed the area. Nevertheless, Hans insisted on keeping an appointment at the laboratory of one of us (J.L.G.) at a time of day when the traffic conditions were still tolerable. The meeting was, as always, a lively one, but, as the snow continued to pile up, we all became increasingly worried that none of us, and especially Hans, would be able to make it to a safe haven. Hans and Lina were scheduled to return to New York by shuttle. It was a major undertaking to break away from the discussions long enough for Hans to allow us to make hotel arrangements at the Bethesda Hyatt, which is over a Metro stop, and see that Lina, who was still at Walter Reed, reached the hotel. Eventually, we dropped Hans at a nearby Metro stop for what should have been an easily maneuvered trip to the Hyatt. Some hours later, a distressed Lina called to determine the whereabouts of Hans. We later learned that the Metro section where Hans was to board had shut down as he was waiting for the train and Hans, of necessity, had improvised by taking a connecting bus to Silver Spring, eventually working his way back on the Metro in the other direction just making the last train connections prior to the shutdown of the entire system. To those of us waiting for Hans, it was an anxious time. Cold, snow, and uncertain travel were elements that could stress Hans' fragile health—as Lina and we appreciated. To Hans, except for Lina's anxiety, it was a matter of small importance and he later said that they rather enjoyed the unexpected stay at the Hyatt.

Some of the visits by Hans became technical sessions. On the occasion of one visit to the Rockville Laboratory, Eric Gowans, who was on sabbatical leave from Adelaide, asked Hans to review the histology of woodchuck specimens that had been prepared for *in situ* hybridization. Hans jumped at the opportunity and, after a polite amount of time, proceeded gently to instruct us on the limitations of our fixation techniques and then devised new ones on the spot; when eventually modified as suggested, we were delighted with the outcome, although the morphology remained only marginally acceptable to Hans.

Often, Hans would use one of his frequent trips to Washington as an opportunity for bringing scientists together whom he thought should be collaborating. One of us (R.H.P.) recalls being called to have dinner with him one Sunday evening in Bethesda, where he was attending a meeting, to be introduced to Dr. D. Keppler, of Heidelberg, who was also attending the meeting. Typically, Hans saw possible associations between Keppler's work on eicosanoids and the fulminant hepatitis of pregnant women infected with hepatitis E virus. Such was Hans' grasp of the field of hepatology that apparently disparate topics found associations in his fertile mind. Hans never let a potential paper go unpublished. One example: research conducted by a young visiting fellow had to do with the histopathology of co-infections and superinfections of two or more hepatitis viruses. Hans, who served as a mentor for the studies, became very interested in the histopathologic characteristics of the superimposed hepatitis in such cases. As often happens, the project dragged on as the young scientist returned to his country of origin and became involved with his new responsibilities. But he hadn't reckoned on the tenacity of Hans Popper. At Hans' insistence, the work was eventually assembled, and successive drafts of the manuscript were written and rewritten by the young scientist, by one of us (R.H.P.) and by Hans. Finally, the paper was published in 1990 with Hans as a co-author, approximately 2 years after his death. Such was his strength of purpose.

Similarly, Hans insisted on bringing to completion separate studies on severe hepatitis in Northern South America and hepatocellular carcinoma in native Alaskans that involved numerous individuals and agencies of the U.S. government. Both sets of studies were eventually published and the literature is richer for them. In all, we shared over three dozen papers with Hans.

Hans was, almost surely, the last individual to understand the liver fully. He was an observer and a chronicler but, most important, a founder of the field of modern hepatology. His experience bridged the field from its classic origins of gross and microscopic anatomy to molecular biology and, remarkably, he understood all of it. In this age of specialization, Hans was a generalist who, somehow, was able to keep up with the current voluminous literature in hepatology and to integrate all of this information into a comprehensive understanding of the liver. Yearly, usually during the holiday season, Hans reviewed the entire primary literature on the liver, a formidable task. Certainly, the broad knowledge base from years of this exercise, coupled with his own experience, enabled him to function so superbly in the presentation of the larger overview of a given subject, or to summarize the scientific contents of so many national and international meetings. Those of us who were rather limited in our experimental approaches came away with a respectful appreciation of broader aspects of liver disease. Through his years of study, Hans had a strong sense of history. When the implications of hepatitis delta virus (HDV) infection on HBV liver disease were first revealed, Hans understood the problems of liver disease etiology in South America and the availability of viscerotomy specimens from long ago. We shared his excitement at the finding that many of these specimens were positive for HDV markers and the impact that this has had on the epidemiology of HDV in the Amazon region, with implications for both yellow fever and HBV vaccination programs.

As revealed in our many conversations, Hans was consumed with the need to understand the underlying mechanisms of liver disease and appreciated the potential contributions that each subdiscipline of science could contribute. He understood the scientific method and the differences between the usual evolutionary process of informational flow and the paradigm shift, as exemplified by the Rizzetto discovery of HDV, on the understanding of liver disease. In his interactions with us and our associates, Hans was the physician, the teacher, and the philosopher, to the very end a leader who challenged us to achieve greater intellectual heights. He was an organizer and a synthesizer in the tradition of the great conductors of music, as well as being a virtuoso player in his own right. Yet, he was self-effacing about his extraordinary abilities, describing himself as "just a morphologist."

In late 1987, we were aware of Hans' failing health. In mid-December, one of us (J.L.G.) received a long and personal call from Hans. On urging, he discussed at length his own "objective" diagnosis of his condition and the suitable treatment. The primary reason for the call, however, was to revisit his concepts about the etiology of hepatocellular carcinoma and the important role that the woodchuck might play in the future understanding of liver carcinogenesis; experiments were proposed and a commitment to pursue this scientific problem was exacted, without much reluctance, we should add. It is difficult to express the feelings at the end of the conversation. It was a sad time, perhaps somber is the better word. Hans was convinced that the woodchuck model would yield important answers; it was the counterpart of other rodent models of chemical carcinogenesis. When Bud Tennant, Cornell University, visited Hans in New York with full-thickness biopsy samples of experimental woodchuck HCC, Hans was ecstatic about the quality of material and the ability to examine liver cancer in the absence of cirrhosis, a characteristic of this model. The model was validated in Hans' opinion, by his subsequent examination of specimens from Yupik Eskimos provided by Anne Lanier, in which, like the woodchuck, cancer developed in the absence of cirrhosis. Eventually, these observations led to the "continuum" concept of HCC. In this call, and certainly similar calls to others at this time, Hans was transferring a responsibility to those of us in the biomedical community who were in a position to obtain important answers. Hans felt some sense of urgency and frustration in that we, collectively, were so close to an important understanding of a basic biologic process to which he had devoted much of his life and in which he would most probably not be a participant.

Thus, Hans left us a legacy, and we think of him frequently. In March of 1988, just prior to his death, we made a sad trip to New York. It was, we suppose, a final expression of our regard for this man for whom we each had genuine admiration. We visited his office at Mount Sinai, filled with memorabilia of his rich life, and talked with Clare about trivial things like the disposition of boxes of slides from us that Hans had retained, all the time each of us knowing that the end was near. We wish he were still here to review slides with us, to discuss new and exciting ideas, and to challenge us to move ahead. Yet, we feel his presence in all that we do and know that he will continue to be a major influence in hepatology for the foreseeable future.

We miss him.

32

Marcus A. Rothschild, New York

Whenever I sit back and think of the times I spent with Dr. Popper and, of course, with Lina, I feel a sense of pride and honor in the relationship that we developed. I remember one of the earliest times that I spoke with Hans. This occurred many years after I had watched and listened to Hans at conferences here and around the world. His accurate comments and his outstanding reviews of widely diverse data were unique. He was never too busy or too tired to partake in detailed discussions with the presenters.

To backtrack a little to our first contact, Hans called me and spoke briefly about a series of liver meetings to be held in Freiburg, and he indicated that he would like me to present, in a few minutes, some of our pertinent data on how tryptophan appeared to influence the production of albumin by the liver. I was excited, of course. I accepted with pleasure, and the meeting was a beginning for me. Hans chose to mention, in his summary, some of the few points I had made, and I had a chance, at that meeting, to thank him in person and to meet, for the first time, Lina Popper. Somehow that brief meeting grew to many more and various associations. Many of these were at the council meetings for the American Association for the Study of Liver Diseases. Here I watched, as we all did, Hans' outstanding ability to dissect a particular issue whether it was scientific or political. He explained his point of view in a decisive fashion but without rancor. His words and actions were the means whereby difficult as well as unpleasant possibilities were resolved or prevented. I began to know him as an individual and as a friend. He often said one of our main purposes was never to hurt another individual in our scientific community or in a more general sense. Many times Hans would emphasize this point. I began to learn more about his scientific thinking and his efforts to ferret out the truth. His thoughts would always be in the future, way ahead of most of us and certainly myself.

As our friendship grew, I began to call Hans about problems concerning the Association as well as to give him a progress report of our own research efforts, and the calls became fairly frequent. I would pick up the phone and there would be, "Mark, Hans here. I am calling to see if we can have dinner together." His next sentence would be, "Speak to Lina—see you then." Further conversation would wait until the evening we had chosen. It was as if Hans and Lina had adopted me, and we would share these wonderful, personal, intellectual, stimulating evenings on a frequent basis—sometimes at their home or sometimes at a restaurant. It was always meaningful. At the meeting in Chicago or council meetings elsewhere, we would sit and talk about topics that appeared to influence the direction our Association was taking.

I remember I was secretary when the concept of the journal *Hepatology* reappeared. I remember sitting with Hans as well as others at Mount Sinai, reviewing possibilities and going over the history of the development of the journal. Providing data on other journal activities and presenting these to Hans as well as to the council in general became one of my pleasant tasks. It is with pride that I look back on this time. The launching of *Hepatology* was a wise move by the council under the strong, effective leadership of Hans.

Finally, as I sit back, again with happiness, thinking about the many times we spent together, I cannot conclude this without a word for Lina, a most gracious, generous, and caring friend; a person whom I have learned to love and respect just as I had learned to love and respect Hans. Of course, I am sorry that Hans is not here today because he would be even prouder of how the Association has grown and how his beloved liver activities are continuing to expand. I consider myself most fortunate to have been a friend of his and to have shared in his personal thoughts. Hans' friendship, his torrent of energy, and his great personal warmth have been and will always be an inspiration to me.

33

William Rutter, San Francisco

Like many other biologically inclined scientists, I had long known of Hans Popper's preeminence in the field of liver biology and pathology and his prodigious publication record. Indeed, in the middle 1960s I entertained the possibility of studying hepatic differentiation and read much of Dr. Popper's book on the liver. I found his comprehensive and scholarly treatment rather daunting. Despite his heavy "classical orientation, he attempted to cover all scientific information (including biochemical) relevant to the liver, and to synthesize the mass of gross and specific observations into biological meaning. This tendency was so strong at times that it took on an almost philosophical or literary quality. I was impressed by this unusual treatise, but our studies never really took off, mostly for technical reasons associated with the difficulty of culturing differentiated hepatic cells *in vitro*. Instead, I turned to the (exocrine and endocrine) pancreas as a vehicle to gain some understanding of the differentiation process.

However, my tortuous course in science brought me back to the liver in the late 1970s. I became interested in the possibility of generating a hepatitis B virus vaccine by mimicking the virus surface antigen structure using DNA technology in heterologous cells (yeast). Eventually, after cloning the surface antigen and other viral genes, I attended an International Congress on Hepatitis in San Francisco to learn more about hepatitis. I was impressed by the existence of a huge number of HBV carriers, and their increased tendency to hepatocellular carcinoma (HCC). I was very interested in meeting Hans Popper to discuss the details of hepatitis B associated pathology in hepatitis and the progression to HCC. When Rudi Schmid introduced us, I was surprised by his looks and demeanor. Not only did he look much younger than I expected, but he acted a generation younger. We spent a couple of hours together—he wanted to pick my brain as much as I wanted to pick his! His interests were obviously not restricted to pathology or the liver. I was fascinated by the range of his interests, his awareness of current concepts and developments in a wide range of subjects relevant to biology. Especially, he had a remarkable strategic, tactical, and dynamic sense of science. In the areas of science I knew best he didn't have a detailed knowledge, of course, and sometimes he got the specifics wrong, but he keyed on the pivotal new developments—the ones that provided new insights. He attempted to stretch their meaning to the limit. Whereas his main experimental tool was the microscope, his main experimental weapon was clearly his facile mind. It was great fun to talk with him because his specific knowledge and background was so different from my own. This complimentarity of interests and his engaging personality and dynamic style led us to meet again and again and again. . . . Eventually we became friends.

I was quite busy leading two somewhat divergent lives, one continuing my longstanding scientific interests, and the other directed to more practical considerations—the development of new preventative and therapeutic strategies through biotechnology. Nevertheless, I found it very rewarding to seek out Hans for advice and for fun. His attendance at a meeting was a significant factor in my decision whether or not to attend.

In addition to the hepatitis meetings, I particularly enjoyed the small meetings sponsored by the Kroc Foundation, as well as National Academy meetings, where it was possible to chat on through the wee hours, exploring the events of the day, and then onward to a range of subjects. We always explored the progress on the HBV vaccine, the molecular biology of the virus, retrovirology, the new developments on gene structure and gene expression, mechanisms of hormone action, especially how receptors work, various signaling pathways, strategies of differentiation, prescribed cell lineages versus more adaptive regulative processes, the role of the matrix, evolution of multicellular functions, etc. His integrative faculties were highly developed; he was always trying to make connections, sometimes between the most divergent subjects. Among the biologists, I would compare Popper's way of thinking (though very different in specifics) to that of George Palade, in biochemistry, to H. Krebs, and F. Lippman, each a remarkable individual in his own right and profoundly important in his scientific field.

I really discovered Hans' power base when I agreed to participate in the famous Basel Liver Week, sponsored by Herbert Falk. We had planned to spend a few days in Switzerland after the meeting. Several thousand clinicians and scientists attended from all over Europe and America. The sessions were focused on the hottest subjects in hepatology and biology in general. It strongly featured Hans' interpretative lectures. Here Popper's leadership and style were evident everywhere; he reigned supremely. Hans had asked me to talk about oncogenic mechanisms involving retroviruses, HBV, and mutated peptide hormone receptors. Obviously, this was an ambitious subject; the talk was long, but I enjoyed myself. I gave the talk as if I were discussing the subject with Hans himself without an audience. I then had to leave directly from the lecture hall to catch a plane for Japan.

Hans was obviously the best liver pathologist around. He could put together a talk on any relevant subject, pulling material from a seemingly inexhaustive library of slides. It was totally amazing to me that he could recognize progressive diseases of a variety of different syndromes from analysis of sectioned material. Yet, I became convinced he could; for me this was the ultimate in the practice of classical pathology. But he also transcended that practice. He always managed to coordinate the data derived from the standard methods with the new methodologies as they appeared. In this way, new findings were enriched by the older information. So often scientists operating within a given era are intellectually bound by the concepts of that period; they discard or are unaware of important previous work. Hans was not limited; thus, his views and his vision were unusual and refreshing.

Hans participated in some way in nearly all of the important pathology experiments with hepatitis B. We wanted Hans to do the cytological analysis correlating liver pathology with the first analysis of free and integrated HBV sequences in the liver and sera of hepatitis B and HCC patients. The situation, however, became complicated, and we carried them out at UCSF with Rudi Schmid and Ed Smuckler, who had just become chairman of the UCSF Department of Pathology. Later, Smuckler succumbed to hepatocellular carcinoma himself; looking back, this was probably caused by hepatitis C. Hans later carried out the pathological analysis of Frank Chisari's HBV surface antigen transgenic animals. How excited he was (as was I) when the mouse livers began to display hyperplasia and subsequently tumors!

One of my greatest disappointments is that Hans was unable to attend the Hans Popper Memorial Symposium in December 1988. I wanted to describe the successful cloning by my colleagues at Chiron of the hepatitis C virus, the agent responsible for hepatitis non-A, non-B. This had been a major project since 1982 and in my opinion was the most difficult cloning project yet attempted. Dr. Popper and I had discussed the non-A, non-B project many times, particularly the evidence that had led him to believe it was an agent unlike hepatitis B (this turned out to be true) and played a possible role in hepatocellular carcinoma (now a likelihood). It was a shame for him to go just then. The next several years would have been both a revelation and a culmination for him.

In spite of his prodigious and distinguished scientific legacy, for me the most remarkable thing about Hans was his own personal saga. Out of the racism of central Europe, and the narrowmindedness, if not bigotry, in the United States came a guileless, ebullient, warm, and endearing person. I am enriched by him and will continue to be as long as I have cognition.

34

Fenton Schaffner, New York

WORD GAMES: A FAVORITE OF HANS POPPER

The task of selecting something to describe from a 40-year association with Hans Popper, first as my teacher, then as co-worker, friend, and father figure, is indeed difficult. Those years were good to both of us, although they were not without their problems. We spent more of our waking hours with each other than we did with our families, and we traveled all around the world together (see Figs. 27 and 28 in photo section).

When Herbert Falk asked Paul Berk and me to put together this volume along with Rudi Schmid, my answer was a reluctant yes because I foresaw the difficulty I would have in being objective and succinct. The theme for each contribution was to be how an interaction between Hans and each of us led to some scientific benefit or learning experience. The theme of my effort is "word games" because it was a sport in which Hans often indulged with several of his co-workers but perhaps with me most of all. This coining of new words or phrases or finding new uses for old ones has led to changes in the language of hepatology (a word that Hans did not like).

Our first collaborative effort was a chapter for an early *Advances in Internal Medicine* (1). The purpose of the chapter was to describe the laboratory procedures then in use to assess the function of the liver. We needed a rubric and, after much discussion, settled on "hepatic tests" as more appropriate than liver function tests. Forty years later, some of our colleagues use our term, more recognize that few, if any, are function tests, but most continue to use liver function tests or LFTs.

We put together a scheme for the coordinated use of the hepatic tests and liver biopsy findings (2). We and many others recognized that both histologic and biochemical features of obstructive jaundice could be present with no mechanical obstruction demonstrable. The word "cholestasis" seemed to us to be an appropriate term to describe the phenomenon with the modifier "intrahepatic" for what we were seeing in methyl testosterone jaundice and in some cases of viral hepatitis and "extrahepatic" for obstructive jaundice. Cholestasis had been used to describe bile stasis in dilated bile ducts resulting from obstruction and the bile stasis in some enlarged gallbladders. Our application of the term caught on rapidly, and today it is widely used to describe clinical, laboratory, or pathologic findings that resemble biliary obstruction. Interestingly, despite our own extensive efforts and those of many investigators all over the world, we are still unsure of the mechanisms by which bile flow stops and cholestasis develops.

While we were writing our book, *Liver: Structure and Function* (3), we found that we needed simple terms for various structures or phenomena. One such structure was the connection between the bile canaliculi and the bile ducts. Several terms had been used, but none appealed to us, so we invented the term "bile ductule" or simply "ductule" in analogy to the renal tubule. This term also became widely accepted, but not until the electron microscope enabled us to investigate the details of this structure did we appreciate some of the functions it has (4). Indeed, this first piece of the biliary system continues to intrigue students of normal and abnormal bile flow.

Almost every co-worker Hans had contributed to the "word games." When Hans Elias worked with him, they searched for a name for the configuration of the hepatocytes in the lobular parenchyma. While the term "cord" had been used for years, Elias taught us to think in three dimensions even though we were working with two-dimensional slices of liver tissues. He was a classicist and liked the term "muralium" (for wall) to which Dr. Popper and the rest of us in the group at Cook County Hospital objected. Hans Popper decided that "plate" was the best descriptive term and that is what it has become, with "limiting plate" being the row of hepatocytes surrounding the portal tract (5,6).

After Hans had moved to New York, he found a young Italian doctor, Fiorenzo Paronetto, who had been working as a fellow in the Department of Medicine. Paronetto joined the Department of Pathology for training in that speciality and he and Hans, along with Victor Perez, began looking at hepatic fibrosis, especially in chronic active hepatitis. A name was needed to describe the periportal reaction that consisted of necrosis, inflammation, and fibrosis and so the term "piecemeal necrosis" was born and was felt to be the lesion heralding the development of cirrhosis (7). The term is widely used even though its relation to cirrhosis is not as definite as we thought.

The "gnomes" are a group of pathologists and internists interested in the nomenclature used in hepatic pathology. Hans was one of the founders of the group and looked forward to the meetings of this self-supported and hard-working collection of colleagues. After they had tried to make order out of the chaos of terminology used in chronic hepatitis by devising the terms "chronic active" and "chronic persistent" hepatitis (8), a task in which Hans played a large role, we realized that a third form was left out and the nomenclature was not anatomic. The terms "portal, periportal, and lobular" hepatitis were suggested (9). Lobular hepatitis implied disease with necrosis scattered throughout the parenchyma for longer periods than the arbitrary 6 months required for hepatitis to be called chronic. Such ongoing lobular disease is persistent, but the term had already pre-empted and was generally accepted as describing inflammation confined to the portal tract. Therefore, chronic lobular hepatitis seemed to be the next best thing, and it is being used today.

Another disease that offered a semantic as well as a pathologic challenge was primary biliary cirrhosis (PBC). As we collected more and more biopsy specimens, we began to appreciate the morphogenesis of the disease and proposed the first staging scheme on the basis of liver biopsy findings (10). The name of the disease was obviously a misnomer, since true cirrhosis was present only in the later part of the course of the disease. Therefore, we proposed "nonsuppurative destructive cholangitis" as a more anatomically accurate substitute. While I believe that most of our colleagues recognize the name and accept the idea behind it, the term is too big a mouthful to be practical and probably nothing will replace PBC.

One of the histologic features of later stages of PBC is vacuolization of hepatocytes around portal tracts for which Hans applied the term "cholatestasis" to distinguish it from cholestasis in the same area, which tends to come later (11). Cholatestasis was first used during the 1960s when we were immersed in bile acid investigations. These studies suggested that the concentration of bile acids rose in hepatocytes during cholestasis to the point where they damaged the hepatocellular cytoplasm, particularly the endoplasmic reticulum. The cellular injury led to the deposition of what appeared to be combinations of phospholipid, cholesterol, and bile acid, perhaps in liquid crystals. The vacuoles did stain with Nile blue sulfate, a specific stain for phospholipid. The term has found limited acceptance, and the idea behind it may yet prove correct.

The cholestasis of late PBC and any other long-standing cholestatic process was called "peripheral cholestasis" in the days before the modern (and very old) concept of the organization of the hepatic parencyma (12). Today, "peripheral" is clearly a misnomer, and it should be replaced by periportal or zone 1 cholestasis.

Some terms were selected for alliteration rather than for strict accuracy. One of these was invented while Hans was looking at liver biopsy slides of Hadziyannis in Greece (13). The rather homogeneous cytoplasm of enlarged hepatocytes in HBsAg carriers was likened to ground glass instead of the more accurate frosted glass. Thus, the name "ground glass" cell was applied, and soon the realization came that these cells were the sites of production of HBsAg as proven immunocytochemically and by immune electron microscopy. Ground glass cell is the term now used by all to describe these cells, which are most numerous in the livers of carriers no longer infectious.

Hans liked to put together words because they sounded good and because he could use them as shorthand in slides that he made and in talks that he gave. Examples are "ductular cell reaction," "bile secretory apparatus," and "committed precursor stage of cirrhosis." None of these gained wide acceptance, but that did not deter Hans. The terms were generally descriptive of morphologic features that, in themselves, were not diagnostic but, when used in describing slides, saved a lot of words.

A few terms were dismal failures. Among these were the terms "regular" and "irregular" cirrhosis to describe micro- and macronodular forms (14). We quickly abandoned these ourselves. A term that probably deserves a similar fate but that is still occasionally used is "submassive" to describe either necrosis or collapse.

As the group working with Hans ventured into the field of molecular biology, some new terms had to be devised. One of these was "hypertrophic, hypoplastic smooth endoplasmic reticulum" (15). Again note the alliteration. This term was soon recognized to be an oversimplification, but whether the concept was correct or not was never established. The idea behind it did stimulate a great deal of research by ourselves and others.

Hans never stopped playing word games. His last effort was with Keppler and the result was NIKE for networks of interacting key events, a first major effort by Hans in the use of acronyms (16). They considered hepatocellular injury "a disturbance of a metabolic network or web, rather than a localized defect in a stepwise pathogenetic sequence." This simple concept integrated biochemical and structural alterations into a dynamic complex in which perturbation of one portion sent shock waves throughout the entirety. Hans felt that modulating the effect of the shock wave on the network may be more effective therapeutically than trying to interfere with one step in the process of hepatocellular degeneration. The concept is intriguing and may serve to explain many of the phenomena encountered in the study of the response of the liver to injury.

The greatest talent that Hans had was his ability to integrate pieces of information derived from many different sources. For this he often needed new terms because the concepts represented new views of what we had been seeing all along. I for one enjoyed the "word games" and I have indeed missed them.

References

1. Popper H, Schaffner F. Hepatic tests. In: Dock W, Snapper I, ed. *Advances in internal medicine,* vol 4. Chicago: Year Book, 1950:357–443.
2. Popper H, Schaffner F. Laboratory diagnosis of liver diseases: coordinated use of histological and biochemical observations. *JAMA* 1952;150:1367–72.
3. Popper H, Schaffner F. *Liver: structure and function.* New York: Blakiston, 1957:777.
4. Sasaki H, Schaffner F, Popper H. Bile ductules in cholestasis: morphologic evidence for secretion and absorption in man. *Lab Invest* 1967;16:84–95.
5. Elias H. Pre-examination of the structure of the mammalian liver: I parenchymal architecture. *Am J Anat* 1949:311–33. II. The hepatic lobule and its relation to the vascular and biliary systems. *Am J Anat* 1949;85:379–456.
6. Popper H. Liver disease—morphologic considerations. *Am J Med* 1954;16:98–117.
7. Paronetto F, Rubin E, Popper H. Local formation of gamma globulin in the diseased liver and its relation to hepatic necrosis. *Lab Invest* 1962;11:150–8.
8. DeGroote J, Desmet VJ, Gedigk P, Korb G, Popper H, Poulsen H, et al. A classification of chronic hepatitis. *Lancet* 1968;2:626–8.
9. Popper H, Schaffner F. The vocabulary of chronic hepatitis. *N Engl J Med* 1971;284:1154–6.
10. Rubin E, Schaffner F, Popper H. Primary biliary cirrhosis: chronic nonsuppurative destructive cholangitis. *Am J Pathol* 1965;46:387–407.
11. Popper H, Schaffner F. Chronic hepatitis: taxonomic, etiologic, and therapeutic problems. In: Popper H, Schaffner F, ed. *Progress in liver diseases,* vol 5. New York: Grune & Stratton, 1976:531–58.
12. Popper H, Schaffner F. Pathophysiology of cholestasis. *Hum Pathol* 1970;1:1–24.
13. Hadziyannis S, Gerber MA, Vissoulis C, Popper H. Cytoplasmic hepatitis B antigen in "ground-glass" hepatocytes of carriers. *Arch Pathol* 1973;96:327–30.
14. Popper H, Schaffner F. Hepatic cirrhosis, a problem of communication. *Israel J Med Sci* 1968;4:1–7.
15. Hutterer F, Schaffner F, Klion FM, Popper H. Hypertrophic, hypoactive smooth endoplastic reticulum. A sensitive indicator of hepatotoxicity exemplified by dieldrin. *Science* 1968;161:1017–9.
16. Popper H, Keppler D. Networks of interacting mechanisms of hepatocellular death and degeneration. In: Popper H, Schaffner F, ed. *Progress in liver diseases,* vol 8. Orlando, FL: Grune & Stratton, 1986:209–35.

35

Peter J. Scheuer, London

I spent a year in Hans' department at Mount Sinai, on leave from my post as a lecturer at the Royal Free Hospital School of Medicine at the University of London. My interest in liver disease started in my student days, and I had already embarked on a doctoral thesis on the effects of Senecio alkaloids on hepatocytes when Sheila Sherlock took up her appointment as professor of medicine at the Royal Free Hospital in 1959. Encouraged by the head of my department, Kenneth Hill, I had planned to spend a year in the United States—BTA ("been to America") was considered to be a most useful postgraduate qualification, as indeed it proved to be—but I had not at first chosen Hans Popper's department in New York. Luckily, I was not accepted by my first choice and was then advised by Sheila Sherlock and others to write to Hans. He agreed to take me, and I was able to finance the year with the help of a traveling fellowship from the British Postgraduate Medical Federation.

I arrived in the Department of Pathology at The Mount Sinai Hospital in September 1962. My first memory is of Hans berating a junior pathologist for planning to play golf on the weekend instead of working. I think life must have been tough for the residents and junior staff and the work demanding. As a temporary member of the department, I myself was under much less pressure and greatly enjoyed my relationship with Hans as well as with all the others. Perhaps my view was biased or is colored by the passage of time, but I saw that year as part of a golden era in the department. Everyone seemed to be highly productive and engaged in research relevant to the same issues—mainly the pathogenesis of various forms of chronic liver disease. The senior staff at that time included Fenton Schaffner (part internist and part hepatopathologist), Tibor Barka, Ferenc Hutterer, and Fiorenzo Paronetto. Manny Rubin was beginning to make his reputation in liver pathology. On the surgical pathology side, Dr. Otani gave me my first insight into the classic German-based tradition of detailed macroscopic pathology; he seemed to use microscopy of tumors as mere confirmation of his naked-eye diagnoses.

Hans asked Tibor Barka to take me under his wing, which he did with great patience and kindness. My original idea for a research project during the year had been to try to induce the formation of lipofuscin pigment in rat lysosomes by means of chronic hypoxia, but this was not successful. Out of this idea, however, arose a series of experiments on copper toxicity, since copper overload was also sometimes associated with pigment formation. Tibor and I loaded rats with copper by means of daily intraperitoneal injections of copper sulfate (Barka, Scheuer, Schaffner, and Popper, *Arch Pathol* 1964;78:331–49). Within a matter of days, ultrastructural changes could be seen in hepatocytes by electron microscopy. These included variation in cell density, swelling of microvilli, disruption of cell borders, dilatation of the endoplasmic reticulum and vacuole formation. These changes were interpreted as expressions of cell edema and degeneration. Liver copper levels were markedly increased. After a period of some 2 weeks, granules of varying electron density began to appear near the biliary poles of the hepatocytes, approximately corresponding in appearance to lipofuscin pigment granules. To our surprise, the degenerative changes began to regress about this time, in spite of continuing copper loading and high liver copper levels. We probably began to appreciate the significance of this finding in the process of discussion, but, characteristically, it was Hans who quickly and clearly summarized the study: the pigment represented an adaptive change within the hepatocyte, enabling the toxic copper to be sequestered in harmless form. In time, I learned to appreciate this particular quality of Hans' as perhaps the most striking manifestation of his genius. He would listen to a group of papers at a meeting with close attention; the rest of us (I at least—I cannot vouch for the others) realized that the papers were of interest, but could not quite formulate our reactions. Hans would leap up and, in a few words, explain why the findings were significant, and how they changed the concept of whatever topic was being discussed. Since Hans was rarely absent from any liver meeting of importance, this meant that we were regularly treated to a reappraisal and updating of our concepts of liver physiology and liver disease, for his understanding went far beyond the conventional boundaries of anatomic pathology. I use the word genius deliberately and with forethought: there are many scientists and physicians who advance their subject by discovery and research, but there are very few who, like Hans, could rapidly and accurately synthesize the results of others with such mental elegance.

What else did Hans teach us at Mount Sinai? His seminars on liver pathology, given weekly to the residents, were lucid, stimulating, and memorable. His comments in the autopsy room showed that he was steeped in the thorough traditions of Austrian and German pathology. His biopsy sessions at other hospitals provided not only a brilliant display of diagnostic skills but also provided an opportunity for hearing those anecdotes of his earlier years for which he was famous. Of the many pieces of advice that he gave me in those months, I will quote only two: write short sentences and specialize in the pathology of one organ! A further statement impressed me and is often recalled now that I am head of a pathology department: "My main job as head," he said, "is to keep my department happy."

My association with Hans grew over the years (see Fig. 29), chiefly because of the "gnomes." This is a group of hepatopathologists and clinicians interested in liver pathology formed in the late 1960s to discuss the classification of chronic hepatitis (De Groote et al., *Lancet* 1968; 2:626–8). The name of the group was given by Sheila Sherlock, who noted that the members were manipulating the nomenclature of liver disease in much the same way that the Swiss bankers—the "gnomes of Zurich"—were thought to regulate the world's finances. Hans was an early and lifelong member. Protestations from Hans that the group was essentially European, while he was American and should therefore resign, were howled down annually by the other members. Over the years, we discussed many topics, ranging from hepatitis through drug reactions and cholestasis to biliary tract disease and forms of hepatocellular necrosis. Whatever the topic, Hans would regularly leap from his chair to formulate a new idea at the blackboard or to demonstrate once more his encyclopedic knowledge of the liver (see Figs. 30 and 31 in photo section). At the end of a hard day's work, he would be the life and soul of the evening's parties and dinners. We could not have done without him.

36

Rudi Schmid, San Francisco
Steven Schenker, San Antonio

Hans Popper, the founder and reigning monarch of modern hepatology, died on May 6, 1988. He was a man of colossal intellect, boundless energy, and encyclopedic knowledge who dominated the field of liver disease for nearly half a century. His fertile imagination and intuition initiated or nurtured many of the field's major scientific advances, and his contributions encompassed all aspects of the liver in health and disease. Investigators all over the world sought his critical judgment because the Popper imprimatur, if granted, conferred scientific credibility to new findings and concepts. As an inspiring and stimulating role model, he endowed countless students, fellows,and coworkers with the intellectual curiosity from which sprang new and, at times, unorthodox discoveries. Under the leadership of this grand master, hepatology developed from a predominantly descriptive discipline to a science based on quantitative assessment of function and structure. As we eulogize Hans Popper, let us ponder his roots and his exceptional human and professional dimensions (see Figs. 32–37).

Hans Popper was born on November 24, 1903, in the midst of the proud, glittering elegance of a decadent Vienna, which was then the capital of the faltering Austro-Hungarian Empire. His father, a prominent physician, moved easily among the city's leading artistic, academic, and aristocratic circles, and this was the milieu in which Hans was reared. As would be expected in an intellectual family in old Vienna, Hans received a classical

Reprinted from *Hepatology* 1989; 9:669–74 with permission.

education based on the twin pillars of Greek and Latin, which he mastered so well that many years later he still was able to coauthor with Hans Elias a scientific article written in Latin! The years before World War I were a happy and carefree time for Europe's privileged—the Golden Times of Vienna, as Hans nostalgically called them—and he thoroughly enjoyed both his exclusive school and the luxury of his family's lifestyle. The Popper family originally came from Bohemia, and the young boy spent many happy holidays with his grandparents in Kralovice, memories which he cherished all his life. (In 1968, during the so-called Prague Spring, he took a few intimate friends on a sentimental visit to this charming Bohemian village, including the house where his grandparents had lived.) But this life of plenty came to an abrupt and dramatic end with the outbreak of World War I in August 1914, when Dr. Popper was called to active army duty. When the war's fortunes turned against Austria, eventually resulting in the disintegration of the Hapsburg Dynasty, life in Vienna rapidly became grim, and the Popper family did not escape destitution and biting hunger. Fueled by calamitous inflation, the misery continued into the early postwar years, but after Dr. Popper's return to civilian life and resumption of his practice, the family's fortune was gradually turned around.

Although the period's economic and political turmoil often interfered with scholarly concerns, the young Hans Popper clearly was one of his humanistic middle school's (Gymnasium) outstanding students, as he was expected to be by his family. He was an intellectually restless young man in search of his personal identity. Toward the end of the war, for example, he passed through a rebellious phase during which he actively fought at the barricades for the despised emperor's downfall, to the understandable horror of his family. His intellectual restlessness accounted for the unusually wide range of academic interests upon which he successively focused attention during his formal education. He decidedly was not a collector or meditator, but rather a dynamic man of vision and action who displayed an almost deterministic attraction to, and fascination with, change, evolution, and progress. It is not surprising that Darwin was one of his lifelong heroes. He was a natural leader whose intellectual dynamism and insatiable curiosity contributed materially to his charismatic personality; these personality traits, however, also explain an aspect of his professional style of which he was quite conscious and which at times bewildered him. As he said of himself, "I jumped too much from one subject to another and thereby missed opportunities which I should have pursued with more perseverance." True, perhaps, insofar as he never succeeded in making a dramatic discovery or breakthrough; rather, his life's work constitutes an almost legendary series of important scientific observations and the positing of novel relationships and challenging hypotheses, provocatively presented, often deeply probing, and always concluding with persuasive, plausible explanations. The total volume and significance of his published contributions are of a dimension and breadth rarely equaled in clinical investigation. And as he mockingly would have added, "Achieved with no other instrument than a light microscope."

In 1922, Hans Popper entered the renowned medical school of the University of Vienna and was instantly seduced by the exciting intellectual environment in which he found himself. His experiences during this time both validated and encouraged his natural intellectual bent for searching curiosity. He was particularly captivated by biochemistry, which, during the postwar years, was emerging as a new and exceptionally promising discipline. As much time as possible was spent in the biochemical laboratory at the expense of attending what were to Hans the unrewarding traditional magisterial lectures. His studies resulted in eight publications, in many of which the student Popper was the first author. Among these, two papers coauthored with Zacharius Dische were particularly noteworthy because they opened the way to quantitative determination of complex tissue carbohydrates.

After graduation from medical school in 1928, the young physician spent his first 5 postgraduate years in anatomical pathology, which then was the conventional path to an academic career in medicine. But he soon became bored with mere descriptive research and established a biochemical laboratory within the pathology service which still exists today, dedicated to Hans Popper. His burgeoning interest in dynamic approaches to pathogenesis naturally attracted him to one of this emerging field's giants, Hans Eppinger, the director of the Allgemeine Krankenhaus' First Medical Clinic, which Popper joined in 1933. Eppinger, a towering visionary, soon became one of Hans' intellectual role models and profoundly influenced his scientific growth and investigative style. Among Hans Popper's most important contributions of this period was the development of the time-honored creatinine clearance test for assessing kidney function. His concepts of renal physiology were quite unorthodox and prompted Homer Smith to remark, "This crazy guy thinks sodium dances a minuet in the renal medulla," a rebuke he later graciously withdrew.

The years at the First Medical Clinic were among the most formative and productive of Popper's academic career but also his most stressful because of the deteriorating political situation. As Germany's might grew, the increasingly menacing Nazi ideology spilled over into Austria, spawning widespread anti-Semitism and eventually leading to the annexation of this small country. In March 1938, when Hitler triumphantly drove into Vienna, Hans was locked up in his office by one of his clinic colleagues. (Ironically, this was the same physician, Lanier, who in 1940 published what he considered conclusive evidence refuting an infectious etiology of catarrhal jaundice.) A few weeks later, forewarned of the imminent danger by a friend, Hans successfully escaped Austria and booked a ticket on the maiden voyage of the New Amsterdam to New York. Aboard ship he came down with hepatitis, but fortunately his jaundice cleared before docking in New York.

His ultimate destination was the Cook County Hospital of Chicago, which a year earlier had offered him a research position carrying a stipend of $250 per month. Although he had declined the earlier offer, now that he was a political refugee he was happy to accept a research fellowship at this busy clinical center for a reduced stipend of $150. He wasted no time in getting his investigations started and took full advantage of the abundant scientific and technical resources at Cook County Hospital. When Hans fled Vienna, Eppinger permitted his favorite student to take with him a used fluorescent microscope, an instrument which was carried to America in Hans' suitcase. It now became a critical tool for his pioneering studies of tissue vitamin A in humans and animals. Andrew Ivy, one of the era's leading experimental pathologists, was so impressed with Hans' ability to identify small amounts of vitamin A in kidney sections that he became one of his closest friends and staunchest supporters. Fluorescence microscopy logically led to the liver, and almost overnight Hans became captivated by liver disease, a common ailment at the Cook County Hospital. As he later said, ". . . and suddenly I was in the liver," a fascination which possessed him for the rest of his life.

The early years in Chicago were a busy time. Hans devoted as many of his waking hours as possible to his new love, investigation of liver injury—experimental, clinical, and pathological. He was particularly intrigued by the pathogenic role of chemical toxins and nutritional deficiencies, such as fat-soluble vitamins and lipotropic substances, in both patients and experimental animals. Among his many scientific reports of this period, the classic observations on vitamin A deficiency-induced liver damage are especially noteworthy. He supplemented his meager stipend by a limited practice of gastroenterology. He soon was joined in Chicago by his father who, incredibly, at the age of 77 had completed an internship, passed the Illinois State Board examination, and started a practice devoted mainly to cardiology. In addition, Hans found time to enroll in the graduate school of the University of Illinois, from which he earned a degree of Doctor of Philosophy in Pathology in 1944.

Hans was initially quite embarrassed that he spoke English with a thick German accent, particularly after December 6, 1941, when his Austrian passport technically made him an enemy alien. Together with a Hungarian expatriate radiologist, he attempted to improve his English skills by enrolling in the Drama Department of the University of Chicago. These studies were abandoned after he heard a lecture by the famous Soma Weiss, professor of medicine at Harvard Medical School, whose strong Hungarian accent clearly had not impeded a brilliant academic career. The Popper accent, both in English and German, became a lifelong trademark about which he and his friends frequently joked because at times it was unclear in which language he was communicating. But communicate he did; his message always came through clear and compelling in any language.

His prolific research work soon resulted in wide scientific recognition and accelerated academic promotion. In 1943, he was appointed director of the Cook County Hospital pathology service and professor of pathology in its Graduate School of Medicine. He also founded and directed the Hektoen Institute for Medical Research, which became an important scientific component of the Cook County Hospital complex. These were exciting times in liver research because fundamental problems of hepatic pathology were at issue, such as the role of alcoholic hepatitis with or without Mallory bodies, and of malnutrition and choline deficiency on the evolution of cirrhosis. Always concerned with mechanisms of disease, Hans made innumerable important contributions to this controversial field, from which gradually evolved the pathogenic concepts, which, having stood the test of time, are currently accepted. The introduction of needle biopsy of the liver, and later of electron microscopy, made it possible to correlate hepatic structure with clinical and laboratory parameters of liver disease. These innovations allowed Hans to recognize and define the syndrome of intrahepatic cholestasis and to identify the early evolutionary stages of hepatic fibrosis. His studies in patients often were backed up by elegantly designed animal experiments, which served as models for human liver disease and permitted the investigation of pathogenic relationships under controlled experimental conditions. Under his imaginative and dynamic leadership, the Hektoen Institute of Chicago soon emerged as a nationally and, after World War II, an internationally recognized center of excellence for research in liver disease, with its director Hans Popper progressively rising to world prominence in hepatology.

Important events also occurred in Hans' personal life during the early war years. On a blind date he met, and later married, Lina Billig, another Viennese expatriate who, with her great emotional strength and sensitivity, exquisite intellect, and Old World charm, became a lifelong partner and compassionate supporter in all of his professional endeavors. Their honeymoon took them to Atlantic City, where Hans had an exhibit at the annual convention of the American Medical Association. Lina helped put up the posters and proudly shared the awarded honorable mention. Two sons, Frank and Charles, were born in Chicago and became the pride and joy of their parents. In late 1943 Hans became a naturalized American citizen and promptly enrolled for active service in the U.S. Army. The Army service, he felt, made him a true American by repaying in some measure his debt to his adopted country. As a commissioned medical officer, it also allowed him to consolidate and expand his expertise in general pathology. He remained a consultant pathologist to the Army until his death and served in this capacity in many important assignments at home and abroad.

After discharge from active duty in 1946, Hans returned to Chicago but decided against resuming his private practice in order to devote all his energy to the pursuit of his scientific interests. True to his dynamic approach to pathology, he focused during these early postwar years primarily on structural–functional relationships in various types of clinical and experimental liver dysfunction, studies which resulted in a much improved appreciation of the values and limitations of available diagnostic laboratory tests. He was also the driving spirit in the founding of the American Association for the Study of Liver Diseases (AASLD), which held its first informal meeting in 1948 at the Hektoen Institute. Attendance was by personal invitation to a small group of Hans' friends who had made major contributions to the nascent field of hepatology. These included William Bean, Jesse Bollman, Richard Capps, Charlie Davidson, Paul Gyorgy, Franklin Hanger, Stanley Hartroft, Frederic Hoffbauer, Robert Kark, Gerald Klatskin, Leon Schiff, Hans Smetana, Fred Steigmann and Cecil Watson. This list is undoubtedly incomplete, because during the AASLD's initial years the annual meetings were quite spontaneous and no records were kept of participants and programs. Papers to be presented were selected by what Hans euphemistically described as deliberate randomness; that is, names were placed in a hat and the requisite number selected in a quasi-blind drawing. Each speaker was allowed 5 minutes and a blackboard for his presentation, which was followed by spirited and often prolonged discussion. In the early years, the annual meetings included a clinical pathological conference featuring cases that had a direct bearing on a controversial aspect of liver disease. These sessions often led to poignant and at times argumentative discussions, including an instance in which the case of a protein-starved rat was presented disguised as the clinical history and pathological findings of a human patient who allegedly had died of severe nutritional liver disease. Hans took enormous pleasure and satisfaction in guiding these annually recurring rites, and under his leadership the AASLD gradually developed into a formally incorporated organization whose annual meetings in Chicago now attract over 2,000 liver experts from all over the world.

As the Western World gradually recovered from the ravages of World War II, Hans increasingly began to reach out to the pathologists in Europe,

South America, and the Far East. In the late 1940s at Yale he met Sheila Sherlock, whose ascendant academic career eventually made her the grande dame of hepatology, and whose lifelong friendship with Hans contributed much to the establishment of a worldwide network of hepatologists. In 1958, this led to the founding in Washington, D.C., of the International Association for the Study of the Liver (IASL), with Sheila serving as its first and Hans as its second president. Other major international meetings took place at the Josiah Macy, Jr., Foundation in New York; at the Ciba Foundation in London; in Havana, Cuba; and in Perugia, Italy, to name only a few of a seemingly endless series of worldwide gatherings of hepatologists, in all of which Hans' unique personal and intellectual qualities made him a natural leader. It was 1957 in Perugia that he met for the first time some of the Continent's leading liver experts, several of whom eventually became his close friends. A group of them, dubbed the "gnomes of Zurich," later met under Hans' leadership in an attempt to develop a unifying classification of chronic hepatitis. This endeavor, despite its perhaps somewhat dogmatic recommendations, had a decisive worldwide influence on the interpretation of hepatic pathology. In 1965, at the Catholic University of Louvain, Hans was awarded the first of a countless series of honors and special recognitions. This was followed by an honorary doctorate from the University of Bologna, which was conferred 3 years after the 300th birthday of Morgagni, whose motto, "Hic locus est ubi mors guadet succurrere vitae" ("Here is the place where death pleases to aid life"), graced his office in Chicago and later in New York. But a recognition of special sentimental value to him was the degree of Doctor of Philosophy *honoris causa*, which his alma mater, the University of Vienna, conferred on him on the 600th anniversary of its founding. On that occasion, he met another renowned honoree, Ludwig Heilmeyer, who in turn introduced him to Herbert Falk, with whom Hans established a deep and mutually rewarding lifelong friendship. It was Hans' personal influence and spirit which persuaded him to sponsor and organize the now-famous, regularly recurring Falk Liver Weeks, which to this day have retained the imprint of Hans Popper's exquisite scientific taste. Over the past quarter of a century, Herbert Falk's generosity and largesse, together with Hans' vision and energy, have contributed immensely to worldwide scientific communication in hepatology.

But it was not all work and science: for example, Hans was a founding member of Chicago's Playboy Club, and in a light moment he was appointed a Kentucky Colonel. He was a refined gourmet who enjoyed a good dinner or party in the stimulating company of his many friends from all corners of the world and was always the gracious center of the event.

In 1957, after Paul Klemperer had retired as chief of pathology at New

York's Mount Sinai Hospital, Hans Popper was recruited as his successor. His arrival in New York had a profound impact on The Mount Sinai Hospital as well as on his personal goals and professional activities. As department chairman in a large academically oriented teaching hospital, he was responsible for a highly rated, extensive teaching program and a demanding pathology service, both of which he directed with his usual brilliance and dynamic enthusiasm. But it soon was apparent to him that to realize the hospital's full potential it needed its own medical school. With persuasive intellect, subtle charm, and unrelenting conviction, he soon won most of his colleagues and the hospital trustees to his plans, and in 1963 The Mount Sinai School of Medicine accepted its first class of medical students. Hans was the architect of the school's curriculum and for years remained its guiding spirit, first as its dean for academic affairs and later as dean and president. He felt that this new school should differ from conventional academic institutions by focusing on three divergent principles: quantitative biology, concern for the individual patient and attention to community needs. Although some measure of success was achieved in each, integration of this troika at times proved difficult, as might be expected when a new medical school is superimposed upon a hospital with a strong tradition of clinical excellence. Hans loved crisis management, and with a combination of diplomatic flexibility and authoritative firmness he usually succeeded in resolving what seemed unmanageable problems.

At the age of 70, he retired from his administrative positions in the medical school and was appointed for life as Mount Sinai's Gustave Levy Distinguished Service Professor. With the reduction in administrative responsibilities, Hans once again was able to concentrate all his energy, curiosity, and enthusiasm on his scientific work, which progressively took on new dimensions, making the final 15 years the most productive period of his life. His stay at the NIH as a Fogarty Scholar brought him into close contact with scientists interested in viral hepatitis. After the identification of the hepatitis B virus in the late 1960s, he was increasingly captivated by the pathogenesis and highly variable morphological and clinical expression of this and other viral infections of the liver. As he said, "In viral hepatitis, the defined factor is the viral exposure, but the completely different outcomes must reflect decisive effects of genetic and/or environmental factors." He was one of the first to postulate the hepatitis B virus' oncogenic potential and to recognize the critical significance of this property for the several hundred millions of viral carriers worldwide. Of equal importance was his realization that investigation and understanding of these problems required familiarity with the concepts and techniques of modern molecular biology, virology, immunology, and oncology. Incredibly for a "retired" professor in his eighth decade, through prodigious reading he acquired this new knowledge with such proficiency that he was able to easily converse and interact with experts in these fields. Said Peter Scheuer,"Hans had the remarkable and genial gift of listening to information from a wide variety of different scientific disciplines and immediately synthesizing it into an updated view of the subject, which he could then transmit to those of us who could think neither so fast nor so clearly." Indelible are the memories of Hans Popper attentively sitting in the front row of international hepatology meetings, seldom leaving the proceedings, and always asking conceptual questions. His comments usually began with a gracious acknowledgement, followed by an analysis of the presented findings with an interpretation often superior to that of the presenter, and at times recognizing the significance of the new information before the author did.

Most of Hans' important, multifaceted investigations of viral hepatitis were carried out in cooperation with scientists of a much younger generation who had been trained in the techniques of modern biology. But he commonly was the initiating and driving spirit of the projects, the one who asked the crucial questions and integrated the new findings into a meaningful concept or hypothesis. Among these were elegant studies of several naturally occurring hepadnavirus infections in animals, which provided conclusive evidence that these hepatitis viruses are oncogenic in the liver in the absence of other environmental carcinogens. Other major contributions concerned the highly variable morphology of non-A, non-B hepatitis and the puzzling biology and pathogenesis of delta hepatitis. He also made the important observation that occupational exposure to monovinylchloride is hepatotoxic, frequently leading to the occurrence of hepatic angiosarcoma.

One of his incidental discoveries was that, unlike other organs, the human liver does not age. This quality of agelessness is an appropriate symbol for the ageless scientist whose lifelong quest was to use current science to make this fascinating organ surrender its secrets. It was this passionate, restless search for new knowledge and his creative imagination, already evident in his youth,which were cited in 1976 when his peers elected him to membership in the National Academy of Sciences, an honor which was among his most cherished.

One may wonder what personal qualities made possible a long life's work of such dimensions and depth. An important element clearly was a brilliant intellect that was shaped, focused, and disciplined by a rigorous classical education in middle school and at the University of Vienna. This kindled his intellectual search for truth and meaning, engendering a lifelong crusade for excellence. He despised mediocrity and demanded from his associates and students long hours of meticulous work, he himself routinely spending 12 to

15 hours a day in the laboratory or library. He was honest with himself to a fault and expected the same from his co-workers. Although he had worked under or with many outstanding scientists and role models, one idol had a particular influence on his scientific career. This was Sir Francis Bacon, from whose writings he learned the importance of the inductive method of science and whose *Essays or Counsels—Civil and Moral,* in its original 1639 edition, was offered him as a gift in recognition of his outstanding services to The Mount Sinai School of Medicine. He also respected his distant cousin, the philosopher Sir Karl Popper, who emphasized the value of formulating a hypothesis that experimentally can be proved right or wrong; any hypothesis that cannot be so proven or that has more than two possible answers was felt to be without merit. He kept a picture of Bacon in his office as a constant reminder of his critical messages.

Decisive as these personal talents and educational experiences may have been for Hans' brilliant scientific career, he himself was fully aware of the old adage that chance favors the prepared mind and prepared his mind was by an unrelenting enthusiasm for his work and an inexhaustible energy that persisted until a few weeks before his death. His life was work and work his life, a personal trait that was graciously accepted and supported by his understanding wife, Lina. But despite his incomparable professional success, Hans remained a warm and generous individual, loyal to and loved by his countless friends, intolerant of arrogance and always prepared to help and support those who were less fortunate than he. Not surprisingly, one of his particular concerns was support of the students and young scientific co-workers in whose intellectual development he took profound interest, and whose stimulating company he greatly enjoyed. There is no greater tribute to this outstanding scientist, teacher, and academic leader than to conclude by quoting the 1974 students' yearbook of The Mount Sinai Medical School:

> Few times in life is one fortunate enough to come to know a man as rare as Dr. Popper. He is a kind and gentle individual, a scholar and teacher who loves learning and who delights in sharing his knowledge with others. He loves life with an exuberance which he joyously imparts to those around him. We feel privileged to dedicate the 1974 yearbook to Dr. Hans Popper.

Acknowledgments: The authors gratefully acknowledge the invaluable support of Dr. Thomas C. Chalmers, Joyce M. McKinney, Clare Dockery as well as Mrs. Lina Popper, who generously gave of her time to provide the authors with background information.

37

Thomas E. Starzl, Pittsburgh

On September 28, 1987, Hans Popper was honored at a convocation at The Mount Sinai School of Medicine of the City University of New York. Many of his friends and colleagues came, and I was asked to give the convocation address. It was a very difficult task for me, since I had so much sentimentality about the subject. I knew, as did everyone there including Hans, that he was dying. He spoke wistfully of a previous distinction that he had received at the same university almost two decades before. He reflected that he had spoken then about how he was in the twilight of his career; he added "now the sunset has arrived." Hans died on May 6, 1988, 7 months later. My remarks about Hans were as follows.

At a convocation in his own university, what can an outsider like me say to Hans Popper who already has received virtually every academic distinction? Hans Popper founded and revolutionized multiple specialties in both medicine and pathology. His pupils learned from him and extended his knowledge and wisdom to every corner of the globe.

Where could this convocation be? There could be many possibilities. In Vienna, where the little boy lived who grew to be a giant and in whose original university the Hans Popper Experimental Pathology Laboratory was dedicated 10 years ago? In Chicago, where Hans moved 49 years ago, one step ahead of a scourge that changed forever the face of his beloved homeland? In his 19 years in Illinois, Hans started over, cared for his family, learned a new language, became professor of pathology at two major universities, and directed the prestigious Hektoen Research Institute. His creativity and productivity were simply prodigious. He became the founder of modern-day hepatology.

Wherever Hans Popper worked, flowers grew, and so it was with Mount Sinai in the New York era: chief of Mount Sinai Pathology, chairman of the Department of Pathology, founding dean, president, and finally the Gustav Levy distinguished service professorship.

I talked to Hans 3 weeks ago while he was in Pittsburgh at an international transplantation conference. In a quiet and solemn conversation, he expressed disappointment at not achieving fully some objectives for Mount Sinai that were dear to his heart. I realized later that these objectives were administrative and, therefore, not even important compared to what Hans had so brilliantly and continuously accomplished in his 30 years in New York City.

Who would deny that institutions are more important than individuals? People come and people go, but in institutions that have a heritage, children of these individuals, their grandchildren, and great grandchildren can fulfill the dreams of future generations. On the other hand, who would deny that the building blocks of institutions are the individuals who spend their lives there? Hans Popper's intellectual legacy to Mount Sinai has been enormous. He brought to it *greatness* of mind and of spirit. Time will not dim the lights turned on here by him or erase the Popper tradition and influence in pathology and medicine.

Once in a while, someone comes along whose position with a university can no longer be described, because his contributions and influence have become universal. Such men and women become more important than all of their jobs, appointments, and job descriptions put together. Then, merely by the act of *being*, they honor the institutions that justly honor them. Cushing of Harvard, Moynihan of Leeds, Blalock of Hopkins. Today, we are honoring Popper of Sinai. A convocation for Hans Popper could be at no other place than at The Mount Sinai School of Medicine of the City University of New York.

My dear Hans, you came to us at a time of tragedy from the crucible of Europe. In this land, you dazzled us with your courage, power, grace, and wit. Our respect for you came early, as you must have known. However, we are here to tell you now, timidly even at this late time, that love from your students, your colleagues, and those who truly knew you was never far behind. Expression of that respect and love is the one true message that I want to deliver today not only to you but also to that charitable and wise woman, Lina, who shared you with us over the years. When I see what you two have done with your lives, I wish I could understand the process. Then, we might be able to make it happen again for others.

38

Frederick Steigmann, Chicago

Walking toward my ward at the Cook County Hospital in Chicago that spring morning in 1938 I was not in a happy frame of mind. I had started to work on peptic ulcer problems with Harry Singer, the gastroenterologist, and Richard Jaffe, the pathologist. Both these men died very young and our plans came to nil. Moreover, my work with Bernard Fantus (professor of therapeutics at the University of Illinois Medical School and director of the Department of Therapeutics at the Cook County Hospital) also suffered when a heart condition prevented his usual inspiring and enthusiastic presence at the research meetings. Then I saw a young man nervously looking around. Having myself experienced many such waits, I asked him whether he was looking for somebody. "Ja, ja. I am waiting for Dr. Arkin." I introduced myself, and he said: "I am Hans Popper and just arrived from Vienna." I asked, "Are you the co-author of *Die Seröse Entzundungen der Leber*? His face lit up: "Ja, ja." I said, "Wunderbar, wunderbar, you are just what we need for our liver studies" and took him to Dr. Arkin. My gloomy mood left me, and I explained to him the general setup in the hospital and at the graduate school where he was to teach. In the days that followed, I helped him to get settled, to meet people, and to set up a private practice. Hans told me that he had brought along a fluorescent microscope, which showed vitamin A in tissues by a green fluorescence and that he was anxious to demonstrate its function. Dr. Fantus had taken a liking to Hans and had promised to help him in his investigations. (For some unexplained reason, the University of Illinois Medical School members were not too excited about his fluorescent microscopic work.) Dr. Fantus, however, was so impressed with Dr. Popper's work that he called him "Hitler's gift to America," a description I have repeated innumerable times.

Thus started our collaboration, the "Hans and Fritz" constellation, which changed many clinical and laboratory procedures at the hospital and helped in the management of patients, especially the ones with jaundice and liver diseases.

I arranged for Hans to meet Dr. Andrew Ivy (Northwestern Medical School), and Hans explained to him the fluorescent phenomenon. Dr. Ivy in turn arranged for Hans to do some blind studies on rats and after he convinced himself that vitamin A could indeed be demonstrated as a green fluorescence in the rat liver, he was helpful in many ways. He sent Hans and me to attend the meeting of the FASEB in New Orleans, where Dr. Popper demonstrated the fluorescence in the livers of vitamin A fed rats and I presented a paper, "Phenolphthalein in Jaundice."

In joining our small liver study group, Dr. Popper gave it a new purpose and direction. We had only the presence or absence of urobilinogen from the urine as indicator of hepatitis (medical jaundice) or (obstructive) surgical jaundice, respectively, and took the increased amounts of urobilinogen as a sign of more severe liver involvement. Hans suggested the use of other biochemical tests for the differential diagnosis of jaundice. A paper, "Differential Diagnosis Between Medical and Surgical Jaundice" (*Am Intern Med* 1948; 29:469), probably best represents our dilemma at that time.

After Hans became part of the group, we attracted more "guests" for our liver rounds, where we discussed clinical data, surgical findings, the few laboratory test results, and at times the surgical and postmortem findings of similar cases. Everyone was thrilled with his explanation of symptoms and findings. Hans was a good lecturer, and the house staff and other visitors enjoyed his presentations despite his heavy accent. As for myself, I felt fortunate to be a co-worker of this man; I respected his general human behavior, his great knowledge, and his photographic mind. I also knew that he would be a good influence in the hospital and thus help in the care of our patients. Dr. Popper showed a sense of warmth, kindness, and respect for whomever he met, the students liked him, and the patients enjoyed his knowledge and personal interest. His scholarship and stamina for work were recognized by all. One of the things that soon became known was the fact that every morning he would go to the library and peruse most of the new journals, a habit that I understand he maintained to the very end. More and more persons from other institutions collaborated in studies performed at Cook County Hospital and, of course, attending men and residents cooperated on some aspects of liver research. Dr. Popper attracted many young coworkers and always insisted that their names be on published papers. He also knew how to choose the right collaborator, e.g., Fenton Schaffner, his lifelong co-worker.

In 1942, we presented a scientific exhibit, "Liver Function Tests in Clinical Medicine" at the AMA meeting in Atlantic City at which we demonstrated the vitamin A fluorescence in normal and its absence in diseased livers. We received a certificate of merit.

It was Hans' goal to make County Hospital a research center. We proposed such a plan to Dr. Karl Meyer (superintendent of the hospital and chief of surgery), who accepted and presented the idea to the hospital board because such a place would give the junior and senior staff the opportunity to do basic scientific research in an orderly and guided fashion. The board okayed it, and in 1943 The Ludvig Hektoen Institute for Medical Research was born as the laboratory facility of the hospital and a place for research and investigation. Dr. Ludvig Hektoen, the "father of pure medical science," had been helpful and supportive, for which Hans was grateful. Various clinical investigations were started, one of them under a government grant, i.e., pectin as plasma substitute; the clinical value, effects, and complications of the different sulfonamides, etc.

In the fall of 1943, Hans earned a Ph.D. in pathology at the University of Illinois. In the spring of the following year, he joined the army and I entered the navy. He spent his time doing pathology and saw a great many cases of hepatitis, quite rampant in the army hospitals. He told me often that this was a priceless experience for him. I served as chief of medicine at the Balboa Naval Hospital in the Panama Canal Zone, where we saw only a few hepatitis cases. Both of us returned to Cook County and quickly restarted the old routine: hospital rounds in wards and the laboratories, respectively, from 8 a.m. to 10 p.m. or later. Hans became the pathologist of the hospital, and the number of laboratory tests on jaundiced patients multiplied.

In the late 1940s and 1950s, Hans, as pathologist of Cook County Hospital, gave brilliant clinical pathological conferences every Thursday at 11 a.m. with standing room only in the amphitheater of the morgue. Most doctors considered this an important learning event. The liver group still had weekly liver slide conferences, and Hans was as involved and cooperative as ever, but the winds of change seemed to be in the air. Meetings, conferences, lectures, e.g., the Macy Meeting, Army Research Council, etc., kept him busy and traveling. Visitors' invitations put demands on his time and knowledge and picked his brain, but Hans never said no.

Dr. Sheila Sherlock had visited Chicago and us in 1947 and invited us to London in 1950 to a liver meeting. Even before that, Hans would talk about organizing a liver society in Chicago. There were no objections from the hospital officials, and our co-workers were enthusiastic. Invitations were sent out for a meeting in the fall of 1950 to meet at the Hektoen Institute.

Agenda: formation of a liver society. Thus, the AASLD was born. We worked hard to make the "liver society" a success. The first eight presidents were easterners who would bring prestige; in later years there was a more even geographical distribution. Hans also believed in the personal touch, e.g., we would take some officers—past, present, and future—to lunch. My co-workers would often describe me as "always the bridesmaid, never the bride." My response was that I was happy to be part of Popper's team and entourage. Gradually, Hans was becoming the liver man with a national and international reputation, and so I finally realized that the constellation of "Hans and Fritz" had disappeared and only a single star, Hans Popper, remained to illuminate the hepatology universe.

After his move to New York, we met at various medical meetings, where he always greeted me with a big "Hello, Fred," but we never had enough time for a real conversation, because his many admirers surrounded him.

The last letter I received from Hans was an answer to my congratulatory note on the establishment of the Liver Foundation Hans Popper Award, in which I stated: "We simple mortals, when aging, console ourselves with the dictum 'sic transit gloria mundi,' but Hans Popper gets more honors and awards as he grows older." It was dated February 11, 1987, and it sums up the lives of Hans and myself for the past 50 years, 18 of which (1938–1956) we spent working closely together in Chicago.

Dear Ruth and Fred,

I received your gracious letter of January 27 and I was deeply moved. You are most kind and even if much of your praise is not deserved, I am of course very pleased to receive it. Thank you.

It was very nice of Fred to write me and it reminds me of the many years we were working together in Chicago and faced many problems and also successes. I am grateful for all the support which I got in these years which also includes Fantus whom you are quoting. I hope you are enjoying your retirement in Champaign and particularly the pleasure of your family. Mine is smaller but what there is, is doing quite well including the two grandchildren.

I am fully retired from almost all diagnostic obligations. Since most recreational activities are not possible for me either for general health reasons or particularly because of my hearing difficulties, I spend more time working in my office than I ever did. This results in some publications but practically nothing is related to co-workers at Mount Sinai. Altogether, I would be most happy if I would feel as well as I apparently look on pictures. Nevertheless we are all trying to go on.

You have in the meantime celebrated your Golden Wedding Anniversary; we were with you in spirit and hope that our letters arrived in time.

With many thanks once more and with best wishes from both of us to both of you.

Sincerely yours,
Hans Popper, M.D.

39

Heribert Thaler, Wien

That the lively baby born on November 24, 1903, one day would become the great Hans Popper is a fact that the medical world owes, not least, to the circumstance that this event took place in the Praterstrasse in Vienna. In those days, Vienna was still the seventh largest city in the world, capital of the great power reigned over by the "old Kaiser," Franz Josef I. Little Hans was once permitted to shake the Kaiser's hand, for a child an exceptional experience, which certainly contributed to the admiration for the noble old man that Hans Popper felt as long as he lived.

Although the threatening signs of decline could no longer be ignored, or perhaps for that very reason, Vienna and with her the whole of old Austria summoned her resources for a golden age of literature, philosophy, art, and science. Otto Friedländer called this period "the last splendor of this fairy-tale city." The intellectual leaders of the epoch were a class of very Austrian, Jewish cosmopolitan intelligentsia. Even after the Imperial and Royal Austrian and Hungarian monarchy had collapsed and Vienna was suddenly only the capital of an impoverished little state, it remained a great power in the intellectual sense. As we know now, much of the intellectual basis of today's world was established then and there in literary cafés and private salons, and Hans Popper was able to participate in his way. Vienna's probably unique golden age of intellect was not to meet its end until it was crushed under Nazi boots.

Hans' father, Karl Popper, was a general practitioner and a highly educated man with considerable foresight. He sent his only child, for whom learning never presented difficulties, to an elite Vienna school, the "Akademische Gymnasium" (academic high school). His schooling completed with honors, Hans decided to follow in his father's footsteps and become a medical doctor.

Vienna was considered at that time to be the Mecca of medicine; its scientific institutes and clinics were almost all filled with world-famous men. It was the end of the great period of the Zweite Wiener Medizinische Schule (Second Vienna School of Medicine): the pediatrician, Clemens von Pirquet, together with the Nobel Prize Winner and discoverer of the blood groups, Karl Landsteiner, established the fundamentals of immunology. The anatomists, Emil Zuckerkandl and Julius Tandler extended the field of functional anatomy, which had been established by Josef Hyrtl. Tandler, who was a pioneering social reformer as well as a teacher, was also a friend of Karl Popper. We owe the classic theory of narcosis to the pharmacologist, Hans Horst Meyer; Sigmund Freud was a colleague of the psychiatrist, Julius von Wagner-Jauregg, who had received the Nobel Prize for the discovery of the malaria therapy of progressive paralysis. Anton von Eiselsberg, successor to Theodor Billroth, founded his famous school of surgery. The orthopedic surgeon, Adolf Lorenz, invented the noninvasive treatment of congenital hip joint dislocation. Ernst Fuchs was the greatest ophthalmologist, probably not only of his time. Of the two radiologists, Guido Holzmeister and Leopold Freund, one invented diagnostic radiology, the other radiotherapy.

Hans passed his preclinical examinations in the shortest possible time and was so brilliant in the anatomy examination that Tandler at once offered him a position as a student instructor. For a student in Vienna at that time that meant not only a salary and financial independence but also a first secure rung on the ladder to success. Thus, Hans was beaming with delight as he hurried to his father and was deeply disappointed to be advised to turn down the offered position and start instead as a laboratory assistant in the physiological chemistry laboratory, whose director at that time was Otto von Fürth, a man famous for his research on vitamins and pigments. Hans trusted his father's far-sightedness and obeyed, although with a heavy heart. At that time, he could not know that this decision would be of such consequence for his later life because, together with pathological anatomy and internal medicine, biochemistry was to become the third pillar supporting his world fame.

At that time, in 1924, a group of young, talented, and enthusiastic doctors were working in Fürth's institute, and Hans made acquaintance for the first time with what today is called a team. The showpiece of the institute's equipment was a simple Dubosq colorimeter. However, at that time, biochemical discoveries still lay about on the streets, as it were. In spite of the primitive equipment, the student, Hans Popper, was able to publish his first scientific papers from this institute, papers that immediately caused no little sensation: together with Warkany he had studied the metabolism of the tuberculosis bacillus. This led to the discovery that this germ can synthesize cyclic from aliphatic amino acids. In 1926, he was able to publish a fundamental work, "Über die Einwirkung von Adrenalin und verwandter Substanzen auf die Selbstgärung der Hefe" ("On the Effect of Adrenalin and Related Substances in the Spontaneous Fermentation of Yeast") in the Berlin journal, *Biochemische Zeitschrift*. Then, together with Zacharias Dische in the same year and in the same journal, the publication of the first nonreductive method for the determination of total carbohydrate content of body fluids and tissues followed. Thus, for the first time, the way was opened for the study of carbohydrates other than glucose and glycogen.

Hans Eppinger, at that time still resident physician with the well-known cardiologist, Karel Friedrich von Wenckebach, knew Hans slightly from this early period in Vienna. Meanwhile, he had been called to take the position of director of the clinic in Freiburg im Breisgau. Now he remembered the diligent and now so successful student and invited him to work for 3 months in his laboratory in Freiburg—a first collaboration that was to have far-reaching consequences.

The next promising event of importance was Hans' examination in pathological anatomy. The astonishing depth of the examination candidate's knowledge moved the director of the institute, Rudolf Maresch, to offer him a position as junior resident. There was, however, a snag: the position was to become available at the end of the year and had to be filled immediately. That was only 2 months away, and Hans still faced his special clinical examinations, 10 in all. Here too, he achieved the apparently impossible: he reported to Maresch with his still-damp doctoral diploma before the end of 1928. His career as a pathologist had begun.

Five years later, Hans' medical career was once again affected by a farreaching change that was triggered this time by an event of historical dimensions. Wenckebach had resigned his position prematurely and of his own free will so that he could concentrate entirely on his studies of the disease beriberi. Eppinger was the candidate at the top of the appointment list. He was, however, not offered the position because of the bitter resistance of a considerable faction of the professorial body who rejected Eppinger because he was reputed to be uncooperative and inconsiderate. Then January 1933 arrived. In the meantime, Eppinger had moved to the clinic for internal medicine at the University of Cologne. Eppinger came from a family of privileged Prague Jews and so, from one day to the next, when Hitler came to power, he was no longer allowed to enter his clinic—he was not, however, at once officially dismissed. In this situation, he telephoned Vienna and made it clear that now was the last chance to offer him the position. Although Austria was at that time still an independent state, the pressure from Germany was already considerable, and it was not possible under any circumstances to appoint a professor who was not tolerated in the German Reich. In this exceptional situation, Eppinger's opponents gave way, although unwillingly, and the appointment took place.

Eppinger was a medical genius and was many years ahead of his time. His influence fertilized the field of internal medicine like that of none of his contemporaries, in particular, the field of hepatology. The classification of jaundice, for example, which goes by the name in America of "Rich," is Eppinger's: Rich became acquainted with it when he visited Vienna.

Eppinger drew his ideas from his work in the laboratories and in the animal house. A totally obsessed experimenter, he might very well have thought even then of testing the validity of his ideas on people, which, however, the high moral standard of the Austrian school of medicine in Eppinger's early years in Vienna did not allow. There is no doubt that one cannot compare the ethical principles of today with those of 60 years ago, but Eppinger went far beyond the limit tolerated even in his day as soon as he was given the chance. This unscrupulousness was his real and decisive character fault and it had to cause his downfall in the end.

Soon Eppinger dominated the medical scene in Vienna and rapidly achieved world fame as a doctor and scientist. Only 2 months after he arrived in Vienna, he remembered the brilliant former student, Hans Popper. The latter had already succeeded in advancing rapidly in the Department of Pathology and now he was offered a transfer to a resident post in the clinic for internal medicine. What that meant must really be explained today: a resident was in charge of a ward and came, in the hierarchy of the clinic, directly below the consultant. Many residents were gray-haired associate professors. Maresch was very unwilling to let Hans go but put no stumbling block in his way because he could not offer him anything equivalent. For Hans, however, he remained a real paternal friend until his death.

Thus, Hans, together with his comrade-in-arms, Hans Kaunitz, who later emigrated to New York, was now in charge of Eppinger's private ward in the "Erste Medizinische Universitätsklinik" (First Clinic for Internal Medicine at the University Hospital). It is clear that life for the two "Hanses" was at first not easy. Their equals in the clinical hierarchy saw them as upstarts and favorites. In addition, the two theoreticians had first to find their feet in the everyday clinical routine. A true story dating from this period still did the rounds in the clinic decades later: In Eppinger's private ward (years later it was to be "mine"), there was a patient with fever. Since they were not able to diagnose its cause, the two wheeled the bed with the patient into a secluded chamber before Eppinger came on his daily rounds. One day, however, Eppinger came unexpectedly early, encountered the removal in the corridor and inquired: "Mr. Popper, where are you going with the typhoid?"

In any case, Hans had now arrived in scientific El Dorado. After a brief flirtation with nephrology, to which he had been animated by Jan Brod, he devoted himself definitively to hepatology. Hans became Eppinger's favorite and his right hand in the clinic's histology and chemistry laboratory. Eppinger's inventiveness and scientific impatience meant that Hans could not spend his days or, more particularly, his nights where 30-year-old, unmarried men are normally attracted. He lived in the clinic and divided his days and often his nights as well between the ward and the laboratory. His parents set eyes on him only on occasional public holidays. But he learned an enormous amount. It was not only his ever-wakeful intellect that came to his assistance but also another gift. W. Kollath said once: "Vieles ist bekannt, aber leider in verschiedenen Köpfen" ("Much knowledge exists but, sadly, in separate heads"). Hans had the rare quality of storing what he saw and heard and finally constructed an edifice of ideas out of the many fragments. No few of the theories that arose in this way have stood the test of later investigations.

Most of Eppinger's scientific publications from his early years in Vienna also carry the name Hans Popper. They include a book [Eppinger H, Kaunitz H, Popper H. Die seröse Entzündung (Serous inflammation). Vienna: Julius Springer, 1935]. It is hardly necessary to say that Hans soon became a good internist to whom even the members of the Vienna professoriate liked to go for treatment. His friendliness and competence won him the respect and, in some cases, the friendship as well of his fellow residents. In addition, it was he who held the courses for Americans in the clinic, which not only brought him considerable financial advantage but also important contacts with "over the water." All this was soon to prove decisive in shaping his destiny.

At the end of 1937 or the beginning of 1938, the Cook County Hospital in Chicago offered him a well-paid position. Hans hesitated to accept because, on the one hand, he had a lot of still unfinished scientific work to do and, on the other, Eppinger had offered to support his "habilitation." ["Habilitation" is the most important step in a scientific career, at least in the countries of the German-speaking world. It requires a large number of scientific publications and a thesis that has to be defended before the assembled professors. Then, if one has also given a satisfactory probationary lecture, one receives the title of "Universitätsdozent" (comparable to associate professor).] Hans already had all the stages of his "habilitation" behind him except for the official presentation by the Austrian federal president when Hitler marched into Austria and, on March 13th, 1939, seized power. Now it was Hans who was to be barred from entering the clinic. Eppinger, of disarming naivity in political matters, was, of course, not a converted Jewish Nazi, as is frequently assumed these days. For him, the Nazis were primitive and bigoted hooligans. As Hans told me later, Eppinger summoned him and said: "Mr. Popper, you had better go home now. In a week the whole fuss will be over; then you can come again!" It was to be a parting forever.

The next days showed that Hans had either a very powerful guardian angel or at least a great deal of luck: his friends made it possible for him to remove his possessions and his scientific papers from the clinic, because Hans did not share Eppinger's optimism. Now he had only to telegraph Chicago to receive by return post the promise of a position, although under considerably less favorable conditions. He booked a first-class cabin on a Dutch ship and intended to have a few pleasant days' holiday in Vienna before leaving. Once again, things did not go according to plan. A friend from the clinic, who maintained the best of relationships with the new rulers, warned him by telephone that he was to be picked up the next morning by the Gestapo. Literally at the very last minute, he managed to obtain a seat on the very last flight that could leave Austria unhindered and so flew, via Prague, to freedom. Hans had become Doctor Popper.

It is futile to fantasize what he would have become had Austria not been engulfed for 6 years by Hitler's "thousand-year empire" and if he had been able to remain in Vienna. Here, too, he would certainly have become a respectable and well-known scientist but never the great Hans Popper. For that development, the "unlimited" possibilities of the United States of America were required and not the all too limited ones of a little state. Thus, in the end even his bad luck brought him good fortune.

Only the capable are lucky or, as Goethe put it much more beautifully in "Faust," Part 2:

Wie sich Verdienst und Glück verketten,
das sehen Toren niemals ein.
Wenn sie den Stein der Weisen hätten,
der Weise mangelte dem Stein.

(How Merit comes to be with Fortune twined
Is to these fools undreamt-of and unknown:
Give them the Stone of Wisdom, and you'd find
Philosophy gone—and what was left, the stone.)

("Faust" translation: Philip Wayne, Penguin Classics, 1959)

40

Hyman J. Zimmerman and Kamal G. Ishak,

Washington, D.C.

We knew of Hans Popper virtually all of our professional lives and had the pleasure of his friendship for many of those years. A particularly memorable phase of that friendship started with his period as Fogarty Scholar at the National Institutes of Health (NIH), when he began to join us at our weekly conferences. Thereafter, on almost all of his monthly visits to the NIH Liver Study Unit, he would join us at the conference—a practice that he continued until his terminal illness.

We knew of him long before that too. When one of us (H.J.Z.) became interested in hepatology at the end of World War II, the Joseph Macy Foundation conferences on liver disease were a rich source of current information. In reading the proceedings of these conferences, the comments that stood out were those of Hans Popper. At the early meetings of the AALSD, Hans was distinctive as a founder of the organization, an enthusiastic and creative discussant, a contributor of important papers, and as the warm host of the cocktail party at the Hektoen Institute of Cook County Hospital, where he was director of the Department of Pathology. When that same one of us moved to Chicago in 1953, he came to know Hans personally and to benefit from his friendship and wisdom and to appreciate his talents in the

168   CHAPTER FORTY

regular domain of his department. The conferences that he conducted (CPCs and "organ recitals") were each a tour de force—and Hans was a strong force in Chicago pathology, hepatology, and medicine and a growing force nationally and internationally in hepatology.

During the quarter-century in New York when he was occupied leading a great Department of Pathology and building an outstanding medical school and leading world hepatology (the "Pope of hepatology," I once heard Rudi Schmid call him), our contact with him was mainly at national and international meetings, which offered opportunities to renew our friendship.

The period that began with his Fogarty Scholarship and regular attendance at our liver histology conferences, occasional attendance at our journal club meetings, and opportunities for more formal exchanges constituted a new era. His enormous knowledge, awesome recall, awareness of new developments and keen histological eye added a new dimension to those conferences. Having started in 1965, the liver histology conference had attained a momentum that became supercharged when Hans joined us. Hans always expressed a never-ending wonder and enthusiasm about the rare and unusual cases that are referred to this Institute in consultation. Often, as he was about to depart, he would say, "Today I learned something new," an expression that vividly summed up his insatiable thirst for knowledge. At one of Hans' visits, we celebrated his 80th birthday (see Fig. 38 in photo section).

There is much more that we could say. From our first look at the hepatology literature (H.J.Z. in 1944, K.G.I. in 1957), Hans' name, like Abou Ben Adam, led the rest. At every meeting of the AASLD (that includes all of them from day 1) and of the IASL, Hans and his ideas predominated, led, and provoked to thought. At the meetings of the "gnomes," Hans led and informed.

His contributions to hepatology, medicine, and medical education are known to all. His friendship and contributions to our lives are inestimable. We appreciated him and will always miss him.

Subject Index